Fit For Life

Your Ultimate Guide To Health, Fitness & Nutrition

Presented by 15 Top Health Experts From Around The World

Fitness Publishing

FIT FOR LIFE: Your Ultimate Guide To Health, Fitness & Nutrition

20 Top Health Experts From Around The World

Copyright © 2023 by Fitness Publishing

Published by Fitness Marketing Group, Sunrise Beach, MO.

Printed in the United States of America

ISBN: 9798861228411

This publication is designed to provide accurate and authoritative information with regard to the subject matter covered. It is sold with the understanding that the publisher is not engaged in rendering legal, accounting, or other professional advice. If legal advice or other expert assistance is required, the services of a competent professional should be sought.

First edition

For more information, contact:

Fitness Marketing Group 182 Oakmont Ave. Lake Ozark, MO 65049

1 (573) 302-8400

Visit us online at: www.fitnessmarketing.com

Table of Contents

Introduction

UNLOCKING THE PATH TO A HEALTHIER YOU

In a world brimming with constant demands and ceaseless distractions, our most valuable possession often takes a backseat—our health. As we navigate the tumultuous journey of life, we often neglect the very foundation that enables us to thrive and conquer the challenges that lie ahead. But what if there was a comprehensive guide, a roadmap to help us rekindle our relationship with wellness, vitality, and lasting happiness?

"Fit For Life: Your Ultimate Guide to Health, Fitness & Nutrition" invites you on a transformative odyssey, one that promises to reshape not just your body, but your entire outlook on life. This book is your compass, your trusted companion in the pursuit of optimal health and well-being.

In these pages, you will embark on a holistic journey that transcends mere weight loss or muscle gain. You'll discover the profound interplay between physical fitness, mental clarity, and nutritional wisdom. Together, we will unravel the mysteries of the human body and mind, delving deep into the science, psychology, and practical strategies that will empower you to lead a life that radiates vitality, strength, and longevity.

At the heart of **"Fit For Life"** are insights from a diverse group of top fitness contributors—renowned experts, athletes, nutritionists, and health enthusiasts who have dedicated their lives to mastering the art of wellness. These luminaries have generously shared their expertise, transforming this book into a treasure trove of knowledge. They have collectively distilled decades of experience and research into actionable advice, ensuring that you have access to the very best guidance on your journey to wellness.

We understand that the world of health and wellness can be bewildering, a cacophony of conflicting advice, quick fixes, and fad diets. **"Fit For Life"** cuts through the noise, offering evidence-based insights and time-tested principles that are rooted in both ancient wisdom and modern science. Whether you're a novice taking your first steps on the path to wellness or a seasoned fitness enthusiast seeking new horizons, this book will meet you where you are and guide you toward your aspirations.

Prepare to embark on a journey of self-discovery, empowerment, and transformation. **"Fit For Life"** is not just another fitness book; it is an invitation to reclaim your health, to uncover your true potential, and to thrive in a world where vitality and well-being are the truest measures of success. Join us on this voyage towards a healthier, happier you, as we explore the profound art of being **"Fit For Life."** Together with our esteemed contributors, we will chart a course to a brighter, healthier future—one where you are the captain of your own destiny, charting a course towards a life that's truly fit for you.

Rick Stret

International Best-Selling Fitness Author

YES YOU CAN: Living An Empowered and Joyful Life Through Fitness

By: Santiago McCarthy

In a world that is constantly evolving and demanding more from us, finding ways to lead an empowered and joyful life has become a vital pursuit. One of the most transformative avenues toward achieving this balance is through fitness. Beyond its physical benefits, engaging in regular exercise has the power to reshape our mindset, boost self-confidence, and infuse our lives with an unparalleled sense of empowerment and joy.

The Connection Between Fitness and Empowerment

Fitness is not just about sculpting your body; it's about sculpting your life. The link between physical activity and empowerment is profound. When you engage in regular exercise, you are taking control of your body and your health. You set goals, overcome obstacles, and push your limits, all of which directly translate to a heightened sense of empowerment in other areas of your life.

The act of breaking a sweat and pushing yourself beyond your comfort zone releases endorphins, the body's natural "feel-good" chemicals. These endorphins not only help alleviate stress and anxiety but also create a lasting sense of accomplishment. This sense of achievement can translate into a newfound belief in your capabilities, encouraging you to take charge of challenges outside the gym.

Cultivating Confidence Through Fitness

A well-rounded fitness routine doesn't just transform your body; it transforms your self-perception. As you witness your strength, endurance, and resilience improve, your self-confidence blossoms. This newfound confidence ripples through every aspect of your life, from your professional endeavors to your personal relationships.

Think about the last time you conquered a challenging workout or achieved a fitness milestone. Remember how that feeling of success lingered long after the sweat had dried? That's the power of confidence gained through fitness. As you set and achieve fitness goals, you are reinforcing the idea that you can accomplish anything you set your mind to, fostering a positive mindset that carries over into all areas of your life.

Finding Joy in the Journey

Embarking on a fitness journey is not just about reaching a destination; it's about embracing the entire voyage. Along the way, you'll encounter small victories, setbacks, and moments of pure determination. Each step of this journey contributes to your growth, both physically and mentally.

The joy derived from fitness isn't solely about the endorphins released during a workout. It's about the sense of purpose and fulfillment that come from prioritizing your well-being. Engaging in physical activity can become an act of self-love and self-care, reminding you that you deserve to invest time and effort into your own health and happiness.

Integrating Fitness into Your Lifestyle

Embracing fitness as a means to an empowered and joyful life doesn't necessitate a radical overhaul of your routine. Instead, it involves weaving physical activity seamlessly into your daily life. Whether it's a morning jog, a lunchtime yoga session, or an evening dance class, finding an exercise routine that resonates with you is essential.

Remember, consistency is key. Small, sustainable changes can yield significant results over time. Prioritize activities that you genuinely enjoy, as this will make it easier to stay motivated and committed. Surround yourself with a supportive community, whether it's a workout group, an online fitness forum, or a friend who shares your enthusiasm for healthy living.

Alright, let me paint you a picture of how easy and awesome it is to weave fitness seamlessly into your daily life.

Meet Sarah, a vibrant and busy bee who's juggling work, family, and the occasional urge to binge-watch her favorite shows. Now, Sarah knows that taking care of herself is a non-negotiable. So, how does she do it?

Morning Energizer: Sarah sets her alarm just 30 minutes earlier than usual. Why? Because she's discovered the joy of a morning workout. Every day, she rolls out of bed, slips into her workout gear, and busts out a quick home workout routine. It's not a marathon, just a series of bodyweight exercises to get her heart pumping and her muscles awake. Not only does this boost her energy levels for the day ahead, but it also jumpstarts her metabolism. Bonus: she gets to check "exercise" off her to-do list before the day even begins!

Lunchtime Liberation: Remember those lunch breaks spent scrolling through social media? Well, Sarah decided to trade them for something more invigorating. She joins a nearby yoga class during her lunch break a couple of times a week. It's a chance to stretch out her body, clear her mind, and return to her desk feeling refreshed and ready to tackle the afternoon. Plus, it's a great way to bond with coworkers who share her newfound love for downward dogs and warrior poses.

Family Fun Time: Sarah is all about quality time with her family. Instead of sitting in front of the TV every evening, they've started a new tradition – evening walks. After dinner, they lace up their sneakers and hit the pavement, exploring their neighborhood and catching up on each other's days. It's become a cherished routine that not only keeps them active but also strengthens their bond.

Weekend Adventure: Weekends are Sarah's playground for fitness exploration. She's always loved the great outdoors, so she's taken up hiking. Every Saturday morning, she grabs her backpack, fills it with water and snacks, and heads to a nearby trail. The fresh air, breathtaking views, and a solid workout make her weekends feel like mini-vacations. Plus, she often invites friends to join her, turning it into a social event that combines exercise with connection.

Dance Like Nobody's Watching: Sarah's guilty pleasure? Dancing like nobody's watching – in her own living room. A few times a week, she cranks up her favorite tunes and lets loose. It's not just fun; it's a fantastic cardio workout that leaves her smiling and energized. She's even started hosting dance parties with her friends, turning her living room into a dance floor and proving that fitness can be an absolute blast.

Supercharging with a Workout Program: One day, while sipping her morning coffee and pondering ways to elevate her fitness journey, Sarah stumbled upon a workout program that piqued her interest. It promised a balanced blend of strength training, cardio, and flexibility exercises – basically, a one-stop-shop for her fitness goals. Intrigued, Sarah decided to give it a shot, and boy, did it take her journey to new heights.

- **Setting Clear Goals**: The first thing Sarah did was sit down and outline her goals. She wanted to build strength, improve her endurance, and enhance her flexibility. Armed with these objectives, she chose a workout program that aligned perfectly with her aspirations.

- **Structured Routine**: With the workout program in hand, Sarah now had a structured routine to follow. Instead of randomly selecting exercises, she had a clear plan for each day. Whether it was a full-body strength workout, a high-intensity interval training session, or a dedicated yoga day, Sarah knew exactly what to expect.

- **Progressive Challenges**: One of the biggest advantages of a workout program is its progressive nature. As Sarah completed each week's workouts, she noticed the exercises becoming gradually more challenging. It wasn't about pushing herself to the limit every time; it was about steady, consistent progress. This approach not only prevented burnout but also ensured that Sarah was continuously improving.

- **Tracking and Celebrating**: Sarah started keeping a workout journal to track her progress. She recorded the number of reps, weights lifted, and even how she felt after each session. This not only allowed her to see how far she'd come but also served as a fantastic motivational tool. On days when she felt less motivated, flipping through her journal and seeing her achievements gave her that extra push she needed.

- **Community and Accountability**: Remember those coworkers who joined Sarah for lunchtime yoga? Well, they jumped on the workout program train too. They formed a mini fitness group, sharing their experiences, challenges, and triumphs. Having friends to share the journey with added an element of camaraderie and accountability that made the whole experience even more enjoyable.

- **Adapting and Evolving**: Over time, Sarah realized that the workout program was more than just a set of exercises. It was a dynamic tool that she could tailor to her needs. If she felt particularly sore one day, she'd opt for a gentler yoga session. On days when she had an extra burst of energy, she'd tackle a more intense cardio workout. This adaptability ensured that her fitness routine remained exciting and suited her ever-changing circumstances.

By incorporating a structured workout program, Sarah not only supercharged her fitness journey but also deepened her sense of empowerment and joy. The program's balanced approach addressed her physical goals while providing a framework for consistent growth. It gave her a roadmap, a community, and a newfound appreciation for what her body could achieve.

If you're ready to take your fitness game up a notch, consider adding a workout program to your routine. Just like Sarah, you'll find yourself on a thrilling adventure of self-discovery, progress, and ultimately, a life that's even more empowered and joyful. You've got this!

See, my friend, integrating fitness into your lifestyle doesn't have to be a Herculean task. It's about finding activities you genuinely enjoy and making them a part of your routine. Sarah's story shows that it's possible to blend exercise seamlessly into your day, whether it's through a quick morning routine, a lunchtime class, family activities, weekend adventures, or just dancing like a superstar.

So, think about what activities light up your soul and get your body moving. Maybe it's a daily walk, a weekly dance class, a weekend bike ride, or even hiking adventure. The key is to make fitness a part of your life that you eagerly look forward to, not a chore to be checked off. And before you know it, you'll be reaping the rewards of a more empowered, joyful, and active you.

The Takeaway

Living an empowered and joyful life through fitness is not an unattainable ideal; it's a tangible reality within your grasp. By engaging in regular exercise, you have the power to transform your body, boost your self-confidence, and infuse every day with a sense of accomplishment and fulfillment. Embrace the journey, celebrate your victories, and revel in the ongoing pursuit of becoming the best version of yourself. YES YOU CAN – and you will – live a life empowered and joyful through fitness.

ele

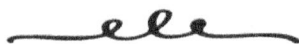

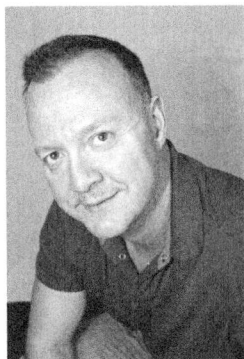

Santiago McCarthy has been coaching private clients towards their goals for over 25 years. As a former martial artist, his passion for fitness is all about movement. Encouraging his clients beyond the concept of a daily workout, he believes in creating customized movement experiences where clients not only look and feel better, but deeply enhance the quality and longevity of their lives. His unique approach and holistic understanding of the body ensures a transformative experience for his clients. His personal fitness regimen varies, but often includes kettlebells, kickboxing, free weights and other high-intensity activity. Santiago's newest book, **"YES YOU CAN: Living An Empowered and Joyful Life Through Fitness,"** goes into much more details and provides the exact blueprint for living the empowered and joyful life you deserve. You can grab his book for yourself at www.successfitnessstudio.com/yes-you-can.

For more information, or to contact Santiago directly, visit info@successfitnessstudio.com.

Rise to Fitness: Empowering Non-Exercisers to Start Strong and Stay Confident

By: Tom Schiltz

Embarking on a fitness journey can be both exciting and intimidating, especially for those who are new to the world of "making their bodies more efficient" (aka... exercise).

The good news is that you're not alone, and with the right guidance and mindset, you can rise to the challenge and achieve your improved health and fitness goals while feeling confident every step of the way. In this comprehensive guide, we'll delve into the essential steps to help non-exercisers kick-start their fitness journey, overcome obstacles, and maintain that newfound confidence. We'll also explore the importance of hiring a coach for personalized guidance and provide insights on navigating a gym setting for a successful and fulfilling transformation.

Step 1: Set "SMART" Goals

"**S**pecific, **M**easurable, **A**ttainable, **R**ealistic & **T**ime bound"

Setting clear and achievable goals is the cornerstone of a confident fitness journey. As a non-exerciser desiring to improve your function, it's crucial to start small and specific. Instead of aiming to run a marathon within a month, consider objectives like walking for 15 minutes a day or completing a beginner's strength and stretching workout routine three times a week. These attainable goals provide a sense of direction, purpose and accomplishment, while boosting your confidence as you achieve them one by one.

Step 2: Embrace the Learning Curve

It's important to remember that everyone starts somewhere, and the initial challenges you face are all part of the learning curve. Embrace them as opportunities for growth and improvement rather than as obstacles. Whether it's struggling with a certain exercise or feeling out of breath during faster movements, each moment of difficulty is a step towards progress. As you become more familiar with different movements and techniques, your confidence will naturally increase, and you'll find yourself mastering movements that once seemed daunting! It happens, I Promise!

Step 3: Find an Activity You Enjoy

The misconception that fitness equates to grueling gym sessions is far from the truth. Fitness is about finding joy in movement and discovering activities that resonate with you. Whether it's dancing, hiking, swimming, or practicing yoga, the options are endless. When you engage in an activity you genuinely enjoy, the workout transforms from a chore into an enjoyable experience. This shift in perspective can significantly impact your confidence and motivation to stay consistent.

Step 4: Build a Support System

No fitness journey should be undertaken in isolation. Building a strong support system can make a world of difference in your confidence and commitment. Whether it's a friend, family member, or an online community, having a support network provides encouragement, accountability, and a platform to share your achievements and setbacks. Sharing your progress and challenges with others who understand your journey can make the process feel less lonely and more rewarding.

I've also seen this inspire other people to begin a better life through exercise journey!

Step 5: Listen to Your Body

As a non-exerciser transitioning into a fitness routine, it's essential to listen to your body and prioritize self-care. Begin at a comfortable pace, gradually increasing the intensity of your workouts to prevent burnout and injury. Rest and recovery days are just as crucial as active days, allowing your body the time it needs to recuperate and rebuild. By practicing self-compassion and honoring your body's signals, you'll build a foundation of confidence that's rooted in holistic well-being.

Step 6: Celebrate Every Achievement

In your journey to fitness, no achievement is too small to celebrate. Completing your first week of consistent workouts, reaching a new personal best, or mastering a previously challenging movement are all victories worthy of acknowledgment. Recognizing and celebrating these milestones, no matter how minor they may seem, boosts your self-esteem and serves as a powerful motivator to continue making you better.

Step 7: Stay Consistent

Consistency is the cornerstone of building confidence and seeing lasting results. Establish a workout schedule that aligns with your lifestyle and commitments, ensuring that you dedicate time to your fitness journey regularly. Over time, as you witness positive changes in your body, energy levels, and overall well-being, your dedication will only strengthen, reinforcing your sense of confidence in your newfound lifestyle.

Step 8: Navigating the Gym Setting

While there are numerous ways to stay active, the gym can offer a structured environment and access to a variety of equipment. Walking into a gym for the first time might be overwhelming, but remember that everyone there was once a beginner too. Familiarize yourself with the layout, ask for a tour, or take advantage of an orientation session if offered. Don't hesitate to approach gym staff with questions; we are more than happy to help.

When using gym equipment, start with the basics. Focus on machines and equipment that target major muscle groups, such as the treadmill, stationary bike, or resistance machines.

Prioritize compound movements over isolation movement to get your biggest bang for your buck.

Here's a sample compound movement workout that targets multiple muscle groups and is suitable for beginners. Compound movements are highly effective because they engage multiple muscles at once, allowing for efficient and effective workouts in a shorter time.

Workout: Full-Body Compound Movement Circuit

Warm-Up (5-10 minutes):

- Light cardio (jogging, jumping jacks, or brisk walking) to increase heart rate and warm up the muscles.

- Dynamic stretches (arm swings, leg swings, hip circles) to improve range of motion.

Circuit: Perform 3-4 Rounds

1. **Squats (12-15 reps):**

- Stand with feet shoulder-width apart.

- Lower your body by bending at the hips and knees, keeping your chest up and back straight.

- Push through your heels to return to the starting position.

2. **Push-Ups (8-10 reps):**

- Start in a high plank position with your hands slightly wider than shoulder-width apart.

- Lower your body by bending your elbows, keeping them close to your body.

- Push back up to the starting position.

3. **Bent-Over Rows (10-12 reps):**

- Hold a dumbbell in each hand, palms facing your body.

- Hinge at the hips, keeping your back straight and core engaged.

- Pull the dumbbells towards your hips, squeezing your shoulder blades together.

- Lower the dumbbells back down with control.

4. Lunges (10-12 reps per leg):

- Take a step forward, lowering your back knee toward the ground while keeping your front knee over your ankle.

- Push through your front heel to return to the starting position.

- Alternate legs for each repetition.

5. Plank (20-30 seconds):

- Start in a high plank position, supporting your body on your toes and forearms.

- Keep your body in a straight line from head to heels, engaging your core.

- Hold the position for the designated time.

6. Deadlifts (10-12 reps):

- Stand with feet hip-width apart, holding a barbell or dumbbells in front of your thighs.

- Hinge at the hips while maintaining a straight back and slightly bent knees.

- Lower the weight down towards the ground, then return to the starting position by standing up and extending your hips.

Cool Down (5-10 minutes):

- Static stretches (hamstring stretch, quad stretch, calf stretch) to improve flexibility and aid in recovery.

- Deep breathing and relaxation to bring your heart rate down and promote recovery.

Notes:

- Perform this workout 2-3 times per week with at least one day of rest in between.

- Use a weight that challenges you but allows you to maintain proper form.

- Rest for 1-2 minutes between each exercise and 2-3 minutes between rounds.

- As you progress, gradually increase the weight or intensity of the exercises.

Remember to consult with a fitness professional or healthcare provider before starting any new exercise program, especially if you're new to exercise or have any pre-existing medical conditions.

Many gyms offer introductory classes or sessions with a Personal Trainer to help you become comfortable with the equipment and develop proper form. These resources can boost your confidence and ensure you're using the gym safely and effectively.

Step 9: The Importance of Hiring a Coach

Working with a coach is a game-changer for non-exercisers embarking on a fitness journey. A coach provides personalized guidance, tailoring workouts to your abilities and goals. They offer expert advice on proper form, technique, and progression, ensuring that you exercise safely and effectively. A coach also serves as a source of motivation and accountability, helping you stay on track and overcome challenges. Our knowledge and experience can empower you to make informed decisions, instilling a sense of trust and confidence in your fitness endeavors.

A coach's role extends beyond the gym; they provide education on nutrition, recovery, and lifestyle adjustments. They customize your fitness **AND** nutrition (after all, nutrition is over 70% of your success equation!) plan to accommodate any limitations or preferences you have, creating a roadmap to success that suits your unique needs. With a coach by your side, you'll navigate potential pitfalls, overcome plateaus, and experience consistent progress, all while fostering a strong sense of confidence in your fitness journey.

Step 10: Keep Learning and Growing

As you become more comfortable with your fitness routine, don't hesitate to explore new exercises and challenges. Trying different activities keeps things exciting and prevents boredom from setting in. This ongoing exploration not only adds variety to your workouts but also boosts your confidence as you conquer new feats. Embrace the opportunity to learn, adapt, and evolve, solidifying your role as a confident and capable participant in your fitness journey.

Conclusion

Starting a fitness journey as a non-exerciser is a rewarding endeavor that holds the potential to transform your life. By setting clear goals, embracing the learning curve, finding joy in movement, building a support system, listening to your body, celebrating achievements, staying consistent, working with a coach, and navigating a gym setting, you'll not only start strong but also maintain the confidence needed to reach your fitness goals. Remember, every small step you take is a step toward a healthier, happier you. Embrace the challenges, celebrate the victories, and let your fitness journey empower you to embrace a confident and fulfilling lifestyle. Rise to the occasion and let your journey to fitness be a testament to your strength, determination, and unwavering confidence. Yes, YOU ARE WORTH IT!

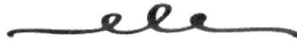

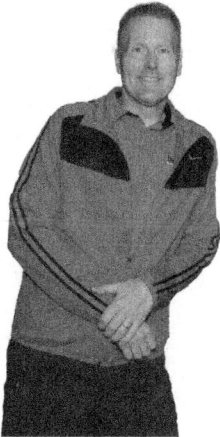

In a world where challenges often come unannounced, some individuals stand out as symbols of resilience and strength. Tom Schiltz is a living testament to the power of fitness and determination.

As he navigated through various stages of life, it became evident that his dedication to physical fitness was not just a hobby but a way of life. Regular exercise, balanced nutrition, and a commitment to overall wellness were the cornerstones upon which Tom's lifestyle was built.

However, it was a fateful incident that truly put Tom's resilience to the test. In 2022, Tom Schiltz found himself facing a life-altering situation—a serious incident that had the potential to shatter dreams and alter the course of his journey. Yet, it was precisely Tom's exceptional level of fitness that played a pivotal role in turning the tide of what was already terribly bad, be much worse.

The incident, which could have resulted in devastating consequences, was met head-on by Tom's well-conditioned body. The physical strength, endurance, and flexibility that had been cultivated over the years became a partial shield against the impact of the incident. Doctors and medical professionals marveled at Tom's ability to withstand the trauma with a level of resilience that defied expectations.

It wasn't just the physical aspect that set Tom apart; his mental fortitude and unyielding determination came to the forefront as he continues his life-long recovery process. The same discipline that had been invested in fitness routines is now channeled into rehabilitation. Every step of progress is a testament to Tom's unshakable willpower.

As a fitness and health professional since 2005, Tom Schiltz has helped hundreds of people achieve their health & fitness goals. His studio and team at *The Fit Stop Fitness Center* motivate clients to reach objectives such as losing weight, toning muscles, strengthening their core, improving mobility and just plain feeling better.

Quite simply, we make your "activities of daily living" easier and more enjoyable... so you CAN do more!

Tom and his team are patient and caring trainers, talking with each client to ascertain their individual goals and develop a customized path to get there. Their passion is, *"Making a difference in people's lives and helping them stay healthy and functional well into the retirement years and beyond."*

Tom is a *Certified Personal Trainer* through the American Council on Exercise (ACE), and holds the sought-after *Functional Aging Specialist* (FAS) credential from the Functional Aging Institute.

Whether you're a beginner or you lead an active lifestyle and need further support, the Fit Stop has a program for you.

Let Tom and his team guide you to a healthier, more functional, and less painful way of living!

info@yourfitstop.com

www.yourfitstop.com

Moving with Purpose: Enhancing Wellness Through Functional Patterns in Daily Life

By: Mike Wilcox

In the hustle and bustle of modern life, the pursuit of wellness, having energy, and living injury or pain free can often seem like an elusive goal, relegated to the realm of resolutions, attempts at quick fixes, weekend workouts, or the belief that "I'm too old" or "I can't do that". However, what if I told you that enhancing your wellness doesn't require drastic measures or hours spent at the gym? By focusing on the positioning and natural movement patterns of your body in your daily life, you can integrate health-enhancing practices into your everyday routine. In this chapter, we'll delve deeper into the transformative power of incorporating a focus on postural positioning in everyday activities such as standing, walking, running, and even throwing, along with a unique approach to increasing flexibility without traditional stretching. All of this will help you unlock the door to a healthier and more vibrant life.

The Power of Standing Tall

At first glance, the act of standing with great posture might seem a bit trivial or an old school phrase your grandparents may have barked at you. However, the truth is that standing well is an underrated hero of wellness. Whether you're waiting for your morning coffee to brew, engrossed in a phone call, or simply taking a moment to reflect, opting to stand with purpose engages a myriad of muscles, including your core, your upper back and leg muscles. This not only improves your posture but also properly aligns the muscles of your body to work for you, not against you. When you are properly aligned, your body moves with grace, it is efficient, and your joints stay healthy and happy. When your body is out of alignment, bad things happen. Muscles end up doing jobs they were not intended to do, thus causing irritation, aggravation, and inflammation, all leading to pain and lots of discomfort.

Imagine the impact of choosing to stand with purpose by adding a little bit of intention throughout your day. Each time you rise from your seat, you're fostering better balance, improving your core strength, and even subtly enhancing your metabolism. Over time, these small shifts accumulate, becoming building blocks for a stronger and more resilient you. And it just takes a little bit of effort and self awareness to create this for yourself. The clients that make the most efficient, impactful progress in our training program are clients who take what they learn in the gym and apply it every day. Hands down, it's easy to see those clients who invest just a little extra outside of the gym to those who do not. It couldn't be more important.

Here's a sample protocol for improving your standing posture using a dowel to perform a few exercises. We often use a dowel (broom stick works very well) or a simple stick to enhance flexibility, mobility, and strength. This protocol focuses on using the stick to promote proper alignment and engage core muscles for better posture.

Protocol for Establishing Great Standing Posture

Duration: Perform this technique for 15-20 seconds at a time, gradually increase the duration as you become more comfortable and proficient.

Equipment Needed: A stick or dowel (about 5-6 feet long).

Standing Posture Technique Protocol:

1. **Stand with your feet right under your hips** (hip width) and knees slightly bent. Hold the stick in front of you perpendicular to the ground, gently pressing it into the floor

2. **Gently 'corkscrew' the floor** with your feet as if you were trying to *"open a jar of pickles."* The goal is to activate your glutes, hamstrings, and outer things. It's the foundation the rest of your body sits on.

3. **Align your hips under your shoulders.** It is typical for hips to be shifted forward, which is not good alignment, causing compression in your lower back.

4. **Find Neutral Lumbar Spine (lower back).** You can do this by tilting your pelvis. Tucking your tailbone 'under' is called posterior pelvic tilt. Lifting your tailbone up is called anterior pelvic tilt. It's important to 'tinker' those two motions until you feel you are in a strong position.

5. **Brace your abdominals** as if someone was going to give you a punch to the stomach. Be sure not to 'crunch' down when doing this. You want to keep length on your abdominal muscles

while contracting them, making them very strong, but also usable (when needed to move).

6. **Extend your thoracic or mid spine**. This is commonly and incorrectly done by solely focusing on lifting your chest or squashing your shoulder blades together. But what you really want to get great at is using your extensor muscles. These are long muscles that run vertically along your spine. These, in combination with your abdominals are key to staying upright, especially as we move.

7. **Pull your chin in**, lengthening your cervical spine or neck. We call this 'chin to throat' and it basically has you giving yourself a double chin. This, coupled with extending your mid-spine is creating length on muscle tissue, thus creating the proper tension your body needs to stabilize your spine.

8. **Firmly press the dowel down** into the floor. The goal is to use the outside muscles of your upper back, your lats, to drive the dowel into the floor. Attempt to lift your ribs away from your hips (we call this elevation or elevating your ribs). You will feel some significant work throughout all the muscles of your body when doing this correctly.

By utilizing these techniques, you now have a scenario where you can develop the body awareness to improve your posture every single day. And this can be done by just practicing for 5 minutes a day. Your legs will become stronger, you will learn that you are capable of using your abdominals to support you, and you will leverage your upper back to stabilize your spine, leading to massively improved movement patterns.

Movements to Improve Your Ability to Maintain Standing Posture While Moving

Duration: Perform this routine 3-4 times per week. Start with a 10-15 minute session and gradually increase the duration as you become more comfortable and proficient.

Equipment Needed: A stick or dowel (about 5-6 feet long).

Warm-Up: Before you begin, spend a few minutes warming up your body. You can do light cardiovascular exercises such as brisk walking or jumping jacks to increase blood flow and prepare your muscles for movement.

1. **Overhead Extension:** Gently hold the stick with a wide grip. Stand tall with your feet hip-width apart. Exhale as you lift the stick over and slightly behind the head, reaching towards the sky. Inhale as you bring the stick back down in front of you. Repeat for 8-10 repetitions. Use the technique #6 above to enhance this movement.

2. **Shoulder Mobility:** Gently, hold the stick with a wide grip in front of you. Keeping your arms straight, slowly raise the stick overhead and then lower it behind your back. Reverse the movement to return to the starting position. Perform 8-10 repetitions. Be careful not to go too far behind your back. Listen to your body and build upon your range of motion over time.

3. **Torso Twist:** Hold the stick horizontally behind your upper back and across your shoulder blades, with your arms stretched out to the side and on the stick. Stand with your feet just outside hip-width. Slowly twist your torso to one side, then the other, while keeping your hips facing forward. This should be done with the abdominals, not the shoulders. To do this, stay braced as you rotate from side to side. Do this slowly at first,

increasing pace as you feel confident your abdominals are dominating the movement. Perform 8-10 twists on each side. Use the elevation technique described in technique #8 above.

Cool Down: After completing the exercises, take a few minutes to cool down and stretch. You could also go for a relaxing walk to cool down.

Tips:

- Focus on your breath during each movement. Inhale deeply and exhale fully as you perform the movements.

- Keep your movements controlled and deliberate. Avoid any jerky or abrupt motions.

- If you experience any pain or discomfort, stop the exercise and consult a fitness professional or healthcare provider.

Remember that consistency is key. Over time, practicing these stick mobility exercises can help improve your posture, increase your flexibility, and enhance your overall standing posture improving how you feel every day of your daily life, while allowing you to take on the daily challenges with confidence and strength.

Step into Wellness: Walking with Intent

Walking, a seemingly mundane action, holds within it the potential to transform your well-being or create chaos in the form of joint pain and muscle stiffness. Instead of considering it merely a means of getting from point A to point B, approach walking as a purposeful practice to keep you strong and capable. Whether you're navigating the corridors of your office, getting outside on a lunchtime stroll, or pacing during an exciting brainstorming session, each step you take contributes to your overall health, positively or negatively.

Humans evolved as walkers, we had to be great at walking to become the humans we are today.. This is how we navigated the world for thousands of years. The last 100-200 years has brought us technological advancements that have humans sitting for far too much of their daily life creating abnormal posture, thus an abnormal walking pattern. In my eyes, this has caused much of the pain the average person has in their daily life. It comes from poor posture. When there is pain, there is much less desire to be an active person and reap all the benefits of being a healthy person. And as I outlined previously, there is much more to posture than just sitting up tall and having a flat back.

Now, in order to walk properly, you first have to be able to stand properly. We established how to do that already. When you stand with proper posture, you have aligned your body, and its muscles to work together efficiently to walk functionally as humans were intended to. Over time, this keeps you from injury, allows you to enjoy activities and live a pretty pain free life!

As an added bonus, walking is a gentle yet effective way to elevate your heart rate, which in turn supports cardiovascular health and boosts your mood. Beyond its physical benefits, walking also provides a unique opportunity to engage with your surroundings, to let your mind wander and recalibrate, and to find moments of peace amidst the daily chaos.

Sample Protocol for Practicing Simple Walking Mechanics

Walking may seem like a natural activity, but practicing proper walking mechanics can enhance your posture, efficiency, and overall comfort. Here's a short sample protocol to help you focus on fundamental walking mechanics:

Focus: Posture and Stride

Duration: Perform this protocol during your regular walks.

Warm-up: Start with 5 minutes of brisk walking to warm up your muscles.

Walking Mechanics:

1. Posture Check (2 minutes):

- Stand tall using the techniques from standing posture protocol.

- Relax your shoulders, letting them sit naturally.

- Engage your core muscles by gently pulling your belly button towards your spine.

- Keep your arms relaxed and swinging naturally by your sides.

2. Stride Length and Pace (5 minutes):

- Take comfortable, medium-length steps.

- Avoid over-striding (taking too long of a step) or under-striding (taking too short of a step).

- Find a pace that feels natural and sustainable for your fitness level.

3. Heel-to-Toe Roll (3 minutes):

- Land on your heel as your foot makes contact with the ground.

- Roll through the middle of your foot and push off from your toes.

4. Hip Movement (2 minutes):

- Allow your hips to move naturally with each step, but avoid excessive swaying.

- Focus on a smooth and controlled movement.

5. Breathing and Rhythm (3 minutes):

- Breathe rhythmically, inhaling through your nose and exhaling through your mouth.

- Match your breath to your steps, establishing a comfortable rhythm.

Cool-down: Finish your walk with 5-10 minutes of slower-paced walking and gentle stretches.

Tips:

- **Mindful Focus**: Throughout the protocol, pay attention to the sensations in your body and how each element of walking mechanics contributes to your overall movement.

- **Practice Regularly**: Incorporate this protocol into your daily walks to develop good walking habits over time.

- **Comfort First**: Always prioritize comfort and avoid any movements that cause pain or discomfort.

- **Gradual Progression**: As you become more comfortable with these mechanics, you can explore more advanced techniques, such as arm swinging and variations in foot placement.

- **Consult a Professional**: If you have specific concerns about your walking mechanics or any underlying health conditions, consider consulting a fitness expert for personalized guidance.

By focusing on these simple walking mechanics, you can transform your daily walks into an opportunity for improved posture, efficient movement, and an enhanced sense of well-being.

Run Towards Vitality

Now, you might be thinking, *"Running? That's for the track and treadmill, not my daily routine. I'm not a runner, why would I need to train for it."* However, integrating running into your everyday movements doesn't require you to pack your running shoes all the time. You don't need to become a long-distance runner to enjoy the benefits of a little bit of running. Consider this: during your walks, infuse short bursts of running, increasing your heart rate and tapping into a wellspring of energy. Alternatively, during moments of downtime, a light jog in place can serve as a quick and invigorating activity as part of your normal exercise routine.

Running, even in these bite-sized portions, offers a wealth of benefits. It enhances cardiovascular health, strengthens your lower body muscles, and releases endorphins – the natural "feel-good" chemicals that can brighten your mood and alleviate stress. By embracing running as an accessible and adaptable activity, you're not just moving your body; you're propelling yourself towards a heightened state of vitality.

A component of movement mechanics that is not talked about in mainstream fitness conversations is what's called elastic recoil. And this is why I think running could and should eventually be a portion of your overall wellness. Elastic recoil happens quite dramatically when running and to a lesser degree, when walking. Elastic recoil is something that is always happening in your muscles. It's essentially the lengthening and contracting of muscles to create movement. One side contracts, while the other lengthens. When running, elastic recoil is working to propel you forward in space. As I mentioned, it is done to a lesser degree when walking, but it is still very important. Otherwise, you would take a stride, pause, then take another stride. It would take you forever to get anywhere! Elastic recoil allows for continuous motion. When done extremely efficiently, you have some of the best athletes in the world. And the reason I am talking about it here is because if we evolved to be walkers/runners, then we evolved to use elastic recoil. Your body actually craves this type of consistent motion to stay flexible, mobile, strong, stable, and active. Thus, running is a great skill to develop to achieve overall wellness.

You can use the same protocol for practicing proper running mechanics as you used for walking. It is important that you listen to your body. When you get tired, your positioning (full-body posture) will begin to be less and less optimal. When this happens, your alignment goes out the door and elastic recoil becomes very inefficient, leading to joint pain and muscle stiffness. Develop body awareness by practicing the standing posture protocol, so that you will notice when your posture slips. When it does slip, you have 2 main options - take a short break or re-align yourself in movement to a more optimal position and continue on.

Throwing: An Unexpected Wellness Boost

As walking was an evolved skill that makes us humans, so is throwing. Early humans had to throw to kill prey, knock things down, break things, and defend themselves. Those who were great at it evolved. The human body evolved to throw. The alignment and biomechanics of the human body require us to take this into consideration when we are training for health, wellness, and longevity. It is an amazing way to train your body to be elastic and fluid and you do not actually have to throw things to gain the benefits of practicing the body mechanics of throwing.

When was the last time you considered throwing as an avenue to wellness? Probably never. While it might not be the first movement pattern that comes to mind, throwing engages various muscle groups and offers a unique avenue for enhancing your well-being. Whether you're tossing a ball with your children, participating in a friendly game of catch, or even practicing targeted throws, you're incorporating a dynamic and engaging element into your routine. This movement pattern is also full of elastic recoil, creating strength, stability, mobility, flexibility, and playability.

The biggest benefit to throwing mechanics is promoting the movement of the spine. Throwing mechanics allows the spine to naturally flex to each side (laterally), extend back, and flex forward all while slightly rotating. **That is amazing if you ask me!** Everyday life is full of movements that require your spine to be great at these things to avoid injury. Throwing mechanics also promote a strong connection from the lower body to the upper body using core strength. I've seen massive strides in my clients upper body mobility and posture by practicing throwing mechanics. It's truly incredible to see the decompression happen and the freedom of movement return in people's bodies. The shoulders, neck, torso, and even the low back and hips loosen up tremendously, become 'unstuck' and decompressed.

The act of throwing can be liberating, allowing you to release tension and foster a sense of lightheartedness that can positively influence your overall wellness. My clients favorite exercises in the gym when they are stressed out are the throwing ones. It is a great feeling to take all your stressful energy and get it 'thrown' out at the gym.

Short Protocol for Proper Throwing Mechanics

Focus: Body Alignment and Follow-Through

Duration: Incorporate these mechanics into your overall training practice

Warm-up: Spend 5-10 minutes warming up your upper body with dynamic arm swings and light shoulder circles.

Throwing Mechanics:

1. Stand in a unilateral stance, hip width, and a walking stride length. (right foot forward and flat, left foot back, heal up).

2. Elevate your ribs away from your hips and slightly rotate your torso to the right.

3. Hold a light object (medicine ball or dumbbell would work nicely) in both hands by your right hip.

4. Lift your left elbow up just above your head, while keeping your hands slightly lower. This will lengthen the muscles of your left side (which you will use to contract in the next step).

5. "Pull" the ball across your forehead as you stride off your right leg, stepping forward, bringing the ball to your left hip. Your left foot is now forward and flat, your right foot is back, heal up.

6. Repeat as you walk forward. Lift your right elbow, 'pull' down and stride simultaneously, bringing the ball toward your right hip.

7. Eventually, with the correct tool (ball), you can start to throw the ball into the floor as you stride and follow through, adding even more benefit to the overall movement.

This sequence has you lengthening and contracting your side muscles, lengthening and contracting your upper back muscles, lengthening and contracting your abdominal muscles, all while flexing, extending, and rotating your spine in a very healthy way. Perfect this little sequence and you will be feeling much less tense and a lot more playable in your upper body!

Tips:

- **Start Slowly**: Focus on proper technique before adding power to your throw. Gradually increase your intensity as you become more comfortable.

- **Consistency is Key**: Regular practice helps reinforce proper mechanics and muscle memory.

- **Target Practice**: Once you start throwing, aim for a specific target right in front of the toes, to improve accuracy and control.

- **Listen to Your Body**: Avoid overexertion and take breaks if you feel strain or discomfort.

- **Seek Guidance**: If you're new to throwing or looking to improve, consider seeking advice from a coach or experienced trainer

Remember, mastering proper throwing mechanics takes time and practice. By following this protocol and focusing on each step, you'll enhance your throwing abilities, whether you're on the field, at the park, or simply enjoying a friendly game with friends.

Increasing Flexibility Without Stretching

While traditional stretching has been a mainstream way to enhance flexibility, there's an alternative approach that can be seamlessly integrated into your daily movements. Functional movements themselves, such as bending, reaching, and twisting, promote flexibility by encouraging your muscles and joints to move through their full range of motion.

As you stand tall, walk with intent, run towards vitality, and engage in throwing activities, you're naturally encouraging your body to explore its flexibility potential. These movements gently coax your muscles and connective tissues to stretch and lengthen optimally, helping you maintain and even improve your flexibility with no dedicated stretching sessions. If you think about it, early humans were not stopping their day to hold a downward facing dog to stretch their hamstrings (the back of your legs). The everyday movements were enough to keep their bodies functioning with flexibility. That is the goal of our training inside of our facility. To develop our bodies to not need to stretch or do a bunch of mobility specific exercises to feel good. We teach the biomechanics of our natural movement patterns of standing, walking, running, and throwing. Throwing, being the deceiving movement pattern most people wouldn't think has much benefit to daily life.

Let's use the throwing technique of lifting the elbow above the head as an example of integrating flexibility into a movement pattern. When done correctly, the side of the body, including the latissimus dorsi (the large muscle on the side of your back) will lengthen creating flexibility in the sides of your body. This movement pattern will naturally improve as you practice resulting in massive flexibility gains throughout your torso. This is extremely important for the proper movement of your spine. The real bonus is as you begin to use more and more of your muscle tissue, you are creating strength and stability alongside your new found flexibility, resulting in massive health gains in ability and confidence.... a winning combination.

Seamless Integration for a Healthier You

The beauty of incorporating natural movement patterns into your daily life lies in its seamless integration. It's not always about carving out additional hours in your day or overhauling your schedule. Rather, it's about making conscious choices that align with your well-being goals, which are also aligned towards longevity. Swap out sitting for standing with purpose during phone calls or brainstorming sessions. Opt for the stairs instead of the elevator and consider a brief jog added to your morning walk. These seemingly minor efforts have the ability to create a more joyful way of life, relieving stress, repairing injuries, and creating a desire to be active, adventurous, filling your life with fun experiences.

Embrace the Journey

Enhancing your wellness through fundamental human movement patterns is not a sprint; it's a meaningful journey towards a healthier, more vibrant you. It's about finding joy in being in control of your body and moving with more purpose. It's about celebrating the fact that your body can move gracefully and without pain. It's also about taking a brief moment once in a while to notice the purposeful rhythm of your steps, the invigorating bursts of running, and the playful arc of a throw. **Each movement, no matter how seemingly small, contributes to the masterpiece of your well-being.**

Embrace this journey with an open heart and a willingness to explore. There's no rush, no finish line to cross. Instead, there's the simple pleasure of feeling your body come alive with each intentional movement. With every step, every throw, every moment of purposeful motion, you're rewriting the narrative of your wellness.

In the chaos of modern life can bring, functional movements are the threads that weave together vitality, energy, and well-being. So, stand tall, walk with intent, run towards vitality, throw in a dash of playfulness in nature, and embrace the inherent flexibility that these movements bring. Let your motions reflect the vibrant and dynamic life you envision. As you embrace these everyday movements with purpose, you'll find that wellness isn't a destination—it's the joyful, fulfilling journey you embark upon each and every day.

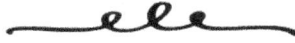

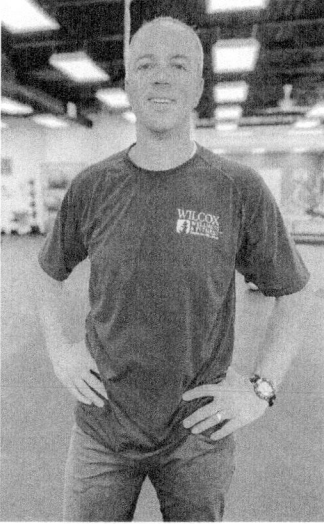

Mike Wilcox, along with his wife, Paige, opened the doors to Wilcox Wellness & Fitness in Bangor, Maine in 2012 and opened a franchise location in Brunswick, Maine in 2018.

Mike loves their business and the impact it makes in the lives of the people we serve.

Mike leads an incredibly passionate team of people who have dedicated their lives to helping others, and he cherishes the opportunity to inspire coaches to be just a little more than they were yesterday.

Mike has dedicated his life to helping his clients become more confident, happy people who are taking life head on & having fun along the way!

As a coach, Mike gets to see incredible transformations in people on a daily basis. This is what motivates him to show up every single day for the last 20 plus years.

After 20 years, he is still amazed at what people are capable of.

These transformations are hard-earned and they come when people fight through their fears, accomplish things they never before thought possible, and as a result, become confident, happy people.

For Mike, there is nothing better than being a part of someone else's success.

There is always a moment in every training session where a client pushes through and does something that they didn't think possible.

Mike lives for that moment.

It is amazing for the client, and it is amazing for Mike and his staff, as coaches.

The mission of Mike and Paige's business is to inspire people to enhance their life by forming helpful habits they can sustain for a lifetime. Mike loves the ripple effect that building healthy habits has in each client's personal life.

Not only do the clients in the program reap enormous benefits, but all the people that their clients come into contact with get to see a confident, happy, and healthy person that hopefully inspires them to invest time and energy in their own life.

When Mike's not working, he loves spending time with his family, traveling, biking, hiking, canoeing, spending time at camp, and being active outdoors.

Mike personally commits to healthy living because he wants to be able to go for a hike at any time, take an active vacation without worry, and play with his kids without fear of injuring himself or embarrassment.

This keeps Mike motivated to maintain his health, his strength, and his endurance.

Mike hopes that he has the opportunity to work with you in the future to help you achieve your health and fitness goals so you can live your best possible life.

Form more information from Mike, or to contact him directly:

Wilcox Wellness & Fitness

PHONE: 207-510-4460

Website: www.wilcoxwellnessfitness.com

Instagram: @wilcoxwellnessfitness

Facebook: Wilcox Wellness Fitness

Fuel Your Fire: Unleash Your Athletic Greatness

By: Seth Scrimo

Welcome to a comprehensive guide that will transform your journey in sports and athletics. Drawing from my experience as a Sports Conditioning Specialist and a Marine Corps Veteran, I'm excited to take you on a transformative journey towards achieving athletic excellence. This guide will delve deep into each of the ten core principles for athletic excellence, providing you with actionable steps, expert insights, and real-world examples to help you reach the pinnacle of your sport.

Principle 1: Unwavering Commitment

Champions are not made overnight, nor is success guaranteed. The first principle on our path to athletic excellence is unwavering commitment. To succeed, you must be "all in," dedicated to your sport, your goals, and your development. The Marines are renowned for their commitment to their mission; similarly, athletes must commit to their training, their teams, and their personal growth.

Let's break it down into the three most essential parts:

Goal Setting for Precision: Think of your goals as the North Star guiding your journey. Start by setting goals that are crystal clear, measurable, and, most importantly, achievable. Whether you're a sprinter, a swimmer, or a soccer player, these goals should resonate with your athletic dreams. Imagine, if you're a sprinter, aiming to shave off 0.2 seconds from your 100m dash time in the next six months. These specific objectives provide a roadmap for your unwavering commitment.

Tailoring Your Training Plan: Now that you've got your goals squared away, it's time to tailor your training plan to match. Break down those long-term goals into bite-sized, manageable chunks. This step is your secret sauce to success because it ensures your daily training routine directly lines up with your big dreams. If you're a sprinter, this might mean mixing in speed drills, strength training, and interval workouts into your daily routine.

Periodization for Sustainable Progress: Here's the secret to going the distance: periodization. This fancy term means organizing your training into different phases, each with a specific focus. Start with building endurance, move on to strengthening those muscles, and finally, gear up for a sprinting-focused phase as your big race day approaches. Why? Because periodization keeps you from overdoing it, allows for the right amount of recovery, and helps you fine-tune your skills to peak at just the right time.

So there you have it! By putting these three friendly, actionable steps into practice, you'll not only commit to your daily training but also set yourself up for a slam-dunk, goal-crushing, success-filled athletic journey. Get out there and show the world what you've got!

Principle 2: The Power of Discipline

Discipline is the bedrock of achievement. It differentiates sporadic progress from consistent success. Like the Marines' unwavering adherence to their code, athletes must follow a disciplined training regimen. Discipline extends to every facet of your life, from nutrition to recovery to skill development. It's the daily habits and choices that mold your journey towards becoming a champion.

Three most crucial steps for building an effective routine:

All-Inclusive Routine: Your routine should encompass not only your workouts but also your nutrition, recovery, and skill development. Think of it as the recipe for your success. Each component plays a vital role in your journey towards excellence.

Stick with It, No Matter What: Commitment is key. Once you've designed your routine, stick to it unwaveringly. Consistency is the foundation of progress. Regardless of circumstances, show up for your scheduled training sessions, meals, and recovery periods. This level of commitment is what champions are made of.

Your Daily Blueprint: Create a daily schedule that prioritizes training, rest, and recovery. This schedule should be non-negotiable, like a critical appointment with yourself. It becomes your roadmap to success. Allocate specific time slots for workouts, meals, and essential recovery moments. These dedicated time blocks will help you maximize your potential and stay on track towards your athletic goals.

By focusing on these three fundamental steps, you'll establish a disciplined routine that sets you on the path to athletic excellence. Commit to it, stay consistent, and let your routine be the driving force behind your journey to success. You've got what it takes!

Principle 3: Embracing Adversity

In both sports and the military, adversity is a constant companion. Champions don't shy away from challenges; they embrace them. It's through adversity that you grow, adapt, and become stronger. Just as the Marines learn to adapt and overcome in difficult situations, athletes must learn to thrive in adversity, using it as a stepping stone to greatness.

The three most crucial steps to embrace challenges effectively in your athletic journey:

Seek Out Challenging Situations: Make it a priority to actively seek challenging situations in your training and competitions. Look for opportunities that take you beyond your comfort zone. This might involve trying new techniques, increasing the intensity of your workouts, or setting ambitious goals. Challenges are the catalysts for growth.

Replicate Competitive Pressures: To perform at your best during competitions, create a training environment that mirrors the pressures you'll face. Here's how:

- **Adverse Weather Conditions:** Train in varying weather conditions to adapt to unexpected challenges that may arise in competition.

- **Simulate High-Pressure Scenarios:** Regularly practice situations that mimic the intensity of real competition, such as match point scenarios or last-minute game situations.

- **Compete Against Tougher Opponents:** Challenge yourself by facing opponents who are stronger or more skilled than you. This will elevate your performance and sharpen your competitive edge.

Gradual Progression: While embracing challenges is vital, do so progressively. Start with challenges that are slightly outside your comfort zone and gradually increase their difficulty. This approach ensures continuous growth without overwhelming you. As you conquer each challenge, raise the bar a bit higher to keep pushing your limits while maintaining a positive and rewarding journey.

By focusing on these three essential steps, you'll develop the resilience and skills needed to embrace challenges effectively in your athletic pursuits. Seek them out, replicate competitive pressures, and remember that each challenge is an opportunity to excel and thrive. Embrace the journey with confidence and determination!

Principle 4: Mental Resilience

Mental toughness is the key to enduring the rigors of both competition and life. The Marine Corps hones mental resilience, and athletes must do the same. It's about staying focused, maintaining confidence, and remaining composed under pressure. Mental resilience is what allows you to perform at your best when it matters most.

The three most pivotal aspects of crafting your pre-competition mental routine:

Visualization: Visualize your success with precision. Imagine yourself stepping onto the field, court, or track and performing at your absolute best. Close your eyes, feel the moment, and vividly picture your movements, surroundings, and triumphant outcomes. This mental rehearsal should be a regular part of your training regimen, helping you engrain success into your subconscious.

Controlled Breathing Exercises: Harness the power of your breath. Implement controlled breathing exercises to maintain composure under pressure. Practice deep inhalations for a count of four, hold for four, and exhale for four. This simple yet effective technique calms your nervous system and sharpens your focus. Cultivate this habit during daily training sessions to make it second nature when competition day arrives.

Positive Self-Talk: Transform your inner dialogue into an unwavering source of confidence. Banish self-doubt and replace it with affirmations like "I am prepared," "I am strong," or "I've got this." During training, keep a vigilant eye on your self-talk, steering it towards positivity and self-assuredness. By consistently nurturing positive self-talk, you'll build an unshakable foundation of belief in your abilities.

These three core elements, when meticulously developed and integrated into your routine, will empower you to face the pressures of competition with the utmost confidence and serenity. Visualize, breathe, and affirm your way to victory!

Principle 5: A Constant Pursuit of Excellence

The pursuit of excellence is never-ending. Just as Marines continually train to maintain their readiness, athletes must maintain their commitment to improvement year-round. This includes refining skills, exploring new training techniques, and seeking guidance from experts in sports conditioning. The relentless pursuit of excellence is what separates champions from the competition.

The three most crucial steps for achieving continuous improvement in your athletic journey:

Continuous Performance Analysis: Frequently scrutinize your performance, leaving no stone unturned. Dive deep into your game, examining technique, strategy, strengths, and areas for growth. Maintain a training journal to track progress and utilize tools like video analysis for detailed insights. This ongoing self-assessment is your compass for growth.

Seek Constructive Feedback: Welcome feedback from coaches, teammates, and competitors. Constructive criticism is an invaluable resource for improvement. Embrace it as an opportunity to refine your skills and adapt your approach. Actively seek out feedback to gain fresh perspectives and identify areas where you can raise your game.

Embrace New Training Techniques: Stay on the cutting edge by exploring innovative training methods, drills, and technologies. Be open to integrating new approaches into your routine. Whether it's revolutionary exercise regimens, mental conditioning strategies, or recovery techniques, adopting innovation can propel your performance to new heights.

By prioritizing these three essential steps, you'll chart a course to continuous improvement in your athletic pursuits. Analyze your performance, actively seek feedback, and remain open to innovative training techniques to unlock your full potential. Your journey to excellence is an ever-evolving adventure.

Principle 6: Teamwork and Leadership

In both the military and sports, the importance of teamwork and leadership cannot be overstated. As an athlete, you're part of a team, and your role matters. Learning to work together, communicate effectively, and lead when necessary are crucial skills. Even individual sports require a team of coaches, trainers, and supporters who play a vital role in your journey.

The three most pivotal steps for excelling as a team player and fostering positive relationships within your athletic community:

Strengthening Communication Skills: Mastering the art of effective communication is the cornerstone of team dynamics. Practice active listening, express your thoughts clearly, and show empathy towards your teammates. Prioritize clear and supportive communication in all interactions, on and off the field. Strong communication builds trust and unity among the team.

Building Positive Relationships: Forge robust relationships based on mutual respect and trust with your teammates and coaches. Get to know your fellow athletes beyond their roles in the sport. Celebrate their achievements and provide support during challenging moments. These bonds create a harmonious environment where everyone can excel.

Embracing Leadership Opportunities: Leadership is not confined to titles; it's a quality that can emerge in anyone. Seize opportunities to lead by setting an example through unwavering commitment, a strong work ethic, and exemplary sportsmanship. Encourage and inspire your teammates to bring out their best. Leadership is about uniting the team and helping everyone reach their potential.

By prioritizing these three essential steps, you'll be well on your way to becoming an exceptional team player and nurturing positive relationships within your athletic community. Elevate your communication skills, build meaningful connections, and embrace leadership opportunities to create a winning team spirit. Your dedication to these principles will set the stage for success, both on and off the field.

Principle 7: Integrity and Sportsmanship

Integrity is at the heart of true sportsmanship. Just as the Marines uphold the highest standards of honor, athletes must do the same. Winning with integrity and losing with grace are signs of a true champion. Sportsmanship not only earns respect but also sets an example for others to follow.

The three most critical aspects of enhancing your sportsmanship and fostering a culture of integrity and respect:

Competing with Unwavering Integrity: Integrity is your guiding principle, both on and off the field. Always prioritize doing what's right, even when no one is watching. Embrace fair play, adhere to the rules, and compete with honor. Whether you win or lose, your integrity remains steadfast, ensuring you're a true champion in every sense.

Demonstrating Respect for Opponents: Your opponents are more than rivals; they're fellow athletes who share your passion for the sport. Show them the respect they deserve. Extend a hand before and after matches, offer encouragement, and acknowledge their dedication. Building a reputation as a respectful competitor elevates the game and fosters a positive environment.

Reflecting and Learning After Each Competition: Each competition is a chapter in your athletic journey. After the final whistle, take a moment to reflect. Analyze your performance, identify areas for growth, and celebrate your achievements. This reflection not only fuels your personal growth but also solidifies the values of sportsmanship within you.

By prioritizing these three fundamental principles, you'll embody the essence of sportsmanship and contribute to a culture of integrity and respect in the sporting world. Compete with unwavering integrity, respect your opponents, and embrace the lessons of reflection and growth. In doing so, you become a true champion both in the game and in life.

Principle 8: Setting and Pursuing Goals

Goals give your journey purpose and direction. Just as the Marine Corps has its mission, athletes must set clear, measurable goals. These goals become your roadmap to success, guiding your training and motivating you to push through challenges. Champions know where they're going and work tirelessly to get there.

The three most pivotal steps to master SMART goal setting for your athletic journey:

Setting SMART Goals: Embrace the SMART criteria to define your goals with precision. Each goal should embody these principles:

- **Specific:** Clearly articulate what you want to achieve. For example, instead of a vague aim like "get faster," specify, "reduce my 5K time by 30 seconds."

- **Measurable:** Ensure your goals are quantifiable. You should be able to track progress in concrete terms, such as seconds or meters.

- **Achievable:** Keep your goals realistic and attainable based on your current capabilities and available time for training.

- **Relevant:** Align your goals with your long-term athletic aspirations. They should contribute to your overall journey.

- **Time-bound:** Set a deadline for achieving each goal, adding a sense of urgency and commitment.

Breaking Goals into Milestones: Transform your larger goals into manageable milestones. These checkpoints serve as progress markers and keep you motivated. For example, if your goal is to reduce your 5K time by 30 seconds, break it into milestones like:

- **Milestone 1:** Achieve a sub-30-minute 5K in two months.

- **Milestone 2:** Record a sub-29:30 5K time within four months.

- **Milestone 3:** Consistently maintain a sub-29-minute 5K time by six months.

Milestones make your journey more tangible and provide opportunities to celebrate achievements along the way.

Regular Goal Review and Adaptation: Remember that goal setting is an ongoing process. Regularly review your goals and assess your progress. Ask yourself if you're on track and if any adjustments are needed. Be flexible and adapt your goals to stay aligned with your evolving capabilities and aspirations. Goal setting should empower you to stay focused, motivated, and in control of your athletic journey.

With these three foundational pillars of SMART goal setting, you'll have a clear and effective roadmap for success in your athletic pursuits. Specific, measurable, achievable, relevant, and time-bound goals, broken down into milestones, and regularly reviewed and adapted, will keep you on the path to continuous improvement and achievement. Your athletic journey is now marked by clarity, precision, and excitement!

Principle 9: Adaptation and Innovation

The world of sports is constantly evolving, and athletes must evolve with it. The Marine Corps values adaptability, and athletes should too. Embrace new training methods, technologies, and strategies. Stay open to innovation and be willing to explore new approaches to improve your performance.

The three most crucial strategies for maintaining a leading edge in your athletic journey:

Stay Informed and Updated: Dive into the wealth of knowledge available in your sport. Stay updated with the latest training methodologies, technological advancements, and strategic approaches. Engage with sports science literature, follow industry news, and immerse yourself in discussions among fellow enthusiasts. Keeping your finger on the pulse of your sport ensures you're always well-informed.

Embrace New Training Methods: Welcome innovation with open arms. Be receptive to exploring novel training methods that promise to elevate your performance. This could involve trying cutting-edge strength and conditioning routines, unconventional mental preparation techniques, or unique skill-enhancing drills. The key is to experiment under the guidance of knowledgeable coaches and experts and integrate what proves effective into your training regimen.

Collaborate with Coaches and Experts: Recognize that you're part of a team, even in your solo endeavors. Collaborate closely with coaches, sports scientists, and experts who have honed their skills over years. Seek their counsel and wisdom to navigate the ever-evolving landscape of your sport. Through these partnerships, you'll gain fresh insights, tailor innovations to your needs, and fine-tune your approach for maximum impact.

By prioritizing these three fundamental strategies, you'll not only remain at the forefront of your sport but also continuously enhance your performance. Stay informed, embrace new approaches, and collaborate with experts. Your athletic journey is now a dynamic quest for excellence and innovation.

Principle 10: Leaving a Legacy

Champions leave a lasting legacy, inspiring others to follow in their footsteps. Just as the Marine Corps' legacy of honor endures, athletes have the opportunity to leave their mark on their sport and inspire the next generation. Becoming a champion is not just about personal success; it's about becoming a beacon of inspiration and leadership.

The three most crucial pillars for effectively mentoring and inspiring young athletes:

Share Your Journey and Wisdom: Your athletic journey is a valuable treasure trove of experiences, both triumphant and challenging. Share your stories, successes, and failures with aspiring athletes. Be open about the obstacles you faced and the lessons you learned. Through personal interactions, blogs, or social media, offer insights that can resonate and inspire. Your authentic narrative can serve as a guide for those following in your footsteps.

Get Involved Locally and Volunteer: Make a tangible impact in your community by actively participating in local sports programs. Volunteer your time as a coach or mentor for youth teams. Your firsthand knowledge can shape the growth of these budding athletes, not just in skills and techniques, but also in the essential aspects of sportsmanship, teamwork, and mental resilience. Being a hands-on role model fosters a direct connection with the next generation of athletes.

Advocate for Inclusive and Supportive Environments: Champion inclusive and supportive environments for young athletes. Promote diversity and encourage an atmosphere where everyone feels valued and accepted. Emphasize core values like respect, fair play, and teamwork. Take a stand against bullying and discrimination, ensuring that sports remain a safe and welcoming space for all aspiring athletes, regardless of their background or abilities.

By prioritizing these three fundamental pillars, you'll become an effective mentor and a source of inspiration for the next generation of athletes. Share your wisdom, get involved locally, and advocate for inclusivity and support. Your mentorship will help shape the future of sports, nurturing not only talented athletes but also responsible, compassionate individuals.

Conclusion

In conclusion, the path to becoming a champion in athletics is not easy, but it is achievable. By following these ten core principles of commitment, discipline, resilience, and integrity, you can chart your course to athletic excellence. Just as the Marine Corps values guide its members to greatness, these principles can guide you on your journey to becoming a true champion in your sport. Embrace them, embody them, and let them lead you to victory and a legacy of excellence. Your inner champion is waiting to be unleashed, and with dedication and unwavering commitment, you can achieve greatness beyond your wildest dreams.

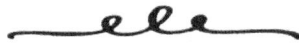

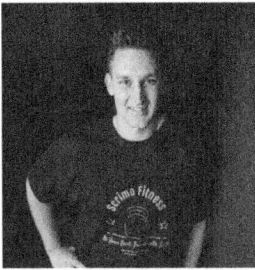

Seth's narrative begins in 2012 when he took a momentous step, one that would set the course for a remarkable odyssey into the realms of health, fitness, and athletic excellence.

Seth's journey unfolded amidst the ranks of the United States Marine Corps. Serving his country instilled an unwavering commitment to discipline, excellence, and the pursuit of physical fitness. These values, imprinted during military service, would become the cornerstone of his future endeavors.

As Seth pursued higher education at Kent State University, his passion for fitness and wellness grew exponentially. Here, he immersed himself in the science of exercise physiology, gaining a deep understanding of the human body's mechanics and the intricacies of peak physical performance.

The culmination of his academic pursuits arrived in 2015 when he graduated with a degree in Exercise Physiology from Kent State University. Armed with this knowledge, he was poised to make a profound impact in the realm of health and fitness.

Seth's commitment to excellence led him to attain multiple certifications from the American Council on Exercise, including prestigious titles like Weight Loss Specialist, Diabetic Coach, and Fitness Nutrition Specialist. However, his journey was far from over. With an unyielding passion for athletic achievement, he ventured into the competitive world of sports conditioning, becoming a certified Sports Conditioning Specialist.

In 2019, Seth recognized the shifting landscape of fitness and wellness, embracing the digital era by completing a certification course through the Online Training Academy. This forward-thinking approach positioned him to effectively guide and support clients in an increasingly remote and tech-savvy world.

Beyond his professional achievements, Seth holds the distinguished honor of being a two-time Amazon bestselling author. His dedication to sharing knowledge and empowering individuals shines through in his literary accomplishments.

Yet, what truly sets Seth apart is his profound understanding of the unique challenges faced by individuals over 30 who grapple with weight-related issues. He has witnessed countless individuals caught in the frustrating cycle of diets and exercise regimens that provide only fleeting results.

Seth's approach is a paradigm shift. It revolves around crafting fitness and nutrition plans tailored to individual needs and lifestyles, making wellness an attainable and sustainable part of daily routines.

But his journey doesn't end with professional pursuits. Seth actively participates in charity races, dedicates early mornings to weight training, and perpetually expands his knowledge through audiobooks. Family is a cornerstone of his life, and he cherishes every moment spent with loved ones. Additionally, he is deeply passionate about mentoring and dedicates his time to the Youth Program at his church.

Aging Gracefully, Training Strategically: Injury Prevention and Functional Training

By Jayson Hunter, R.D., CPT

As the pages of our life story turn, so too do the chapters of our athletic journey. In this pivotal chapter, we explore the art of aging gracefully through the lens of strategic training and injury prevention. Embracing the concept of functional training, we delve into the methods that not only preserve our physical vitality but also empower us to continue our athletic pursuits with passion and resilience.

The Dance of Time and Training

Life after 35 is a journey characterized by accumulated wisdom and a body that reflects the beauty of experience. While the enthusiasm for sports and athleticism remains undiminished, the approach to training must evolve. It's a delicate dance between pushing boundaries and respecting the body's changing needs.

Functional training emerges as a key partner in this dance. Unlike traditional, isolated exercises, functional training hones in on movements that replicate real-life actions. These holistic movements bolster our body's interconnectedness, enhancing strength, balance, and coordination—essential components of injury prevention.

Unpacking Functional Training

At the heart of functional training lies the principle of addressing the body as a whole. Gone are the days of focusing solely on bicep curls and leg presses. Instead, we integrate movements that engage multiple muscle groups and challenge the body's stability.

Imagine exercises like kettlebell swings, which demand coordinated effort from the legs, hips, core, and arms. Picture squats with medicine balls that not only build leg strength but also cultivate balance. These exercises not only promote functional strength but also foster agility, a trait that becomes increasingly important as we age.

Unpacking Functional Training: Elevating Your Athletic Arsenal

In the symphony of aging gracefully and training strategically, functional training takes center stage as the crescendo that harmonizes physicality and longevity. This transformative approach transcends the conventional paradigm of isolated exercises and ushers in a new era of movement-based training that resonates with the rhythms of real life.

The Philosophy in Motion

Functional training rests on a fundamental principle: training movements, not muscles. It aligns with the reality that our daily lives require multi-dimensional movements that engage various muscle groups in synchrony. Whether lifting groceries, chasing after kids, or navigating uneven terrain, our bodies rely on intricate coordination that transcends individual muscles.

The Essential Elements of Functional Training

- **Multi-Planar Movements**: Traditional gym exercises often occur in a single plane of motion. Functional training introduces multi-planar movements that challenge our bodies along various angles and directions. This diversity mirrors the complexities of real-world activities, enhancing overall balance and agility.

- **Core Integration**: Core muscles act as the powerhouse of functional movement. Strengthening these muscles goes beyond achieving the coveted six-pack; it's about cultivating stability that supports every motion, from twisting to lifting.

- **Dynamic Balance**: Functional training emphasizes proprioception—our body's awareness of its position in space. Exercises that challenge balance, such as single-leg squats and unstable surface movements, strengthen neuromuscular connections, reducing the likelihood of falls.

- **Full-Body Coordination**: Movements like kettlebell swings, medicine ball slams, and agility ladder drills engage multiple muscle groups in a coordinated symphony. This holistic engagement mimics real-life activities, enhancing overall functional strength.

- **Joint Mobility and Flexibility**: Integrating mobility exercises and dynamic stretches preserves joint health, counteracting the stiffness that often accompanies aging. A supple body not only reduces injury risk but also contributes to enhanced athletic performance.

- **Adaptability**: Functional training is inherently adaptable. It can cater to athletes of varying fitness levels and can be customized to address specific goals, whether that's improving mobility, enhancing strength, or preventing injuries.

Sample Functional Training Workout: Movement Melody for Injury Prevention

Warm-up:

- 5 minutes of brisk walking or light jogging to elevate heart rate and increase blood flow.

- Dynamic stretches like leg swings, arm circles, and hip circles to promote joint mobility.

Workout:

- **Squat to Overhead Press**: Hold a dumbbell or kettlebell at shoulder height. Perform a deep squat and as you rise, press the weight overhead. This compound movement engages legs, core, and shoulders.

- **Plank Row**: Start in a plank position with a dumbbell in each hand. Alternately row one dumbbell to your hip while maintaining a stable plank. This exercise enhances core strength and stabilizes the shoulders.

- **Lateral Lunges with Medicine Ball Twist**: Hold a medicine ball close to your chest. Step laterally into a lunge, then twist your torso towards the leading leg. This combination enhances lower body strength and core mobility.

- **Single-Leg Deadlift**: Holding a dumbbell in one hand, hinge at the hips and lift one leg behind you. Lower the dumbbell towards the ground as you lift the leg, maintaining a straight line from head to heel. This exercise enhances balance and targets the hamstrings.

- **Bear Crawl**: Get on all fours, with your hands under your shoulders and knees under your hips. Lift your knees slightly off the ground and "crawl" forward, moving opposite limbs together. This primal movement engages the entire body, promoting coordination and stability.

Cool-down: 5-10 minutes of static stretches, focusing on the major muscle groups targeted during the workout. Include stretches for the hamstrings, quadriceps, hip flexors, chest, and shoulders.

Functional training isn't just an exercise routine; it's a transformative approach that empowers athletes over 35 to embrace movement with renewed vigor and purpose. By unpacking its core philosophy and integrating its principles into our workouts, we construct a solid foundation that supports both our athletic endeavors and our journey towards graceful aging. As we lace up our shoes, we embark on a path where each movement echoes our commitment to vitality, strength, and the joy of moving through life's chapters.

The Shield of Injury Prevention

Injury prevention becomes an inseparable companion in our athletic journey. As we gracefully age, our bodies may require more time to recover, and we become susceptible to wear and tear. But this doesn't mean we must surrender to limitations.

Functional training acts as a shield against injuries. The emphasis on balance and core strength, for instance, fortifies the body's foundation, reducing the risk of falls and fractures. The integration of flexibility and range of motion exercises maintains joint health and combats stiffness. This proactive approach is an investment in our athletic longevity.

The Shield of Injury Prevention: Preserving Your Athletic Journey

In the chronicle of athletes over 35, injury prevention emerges as a vital chapter—one that safeguards our ability to participate in the sports we cherish while respecting the shifts that come with age. As we delve into this chapter, we unveil the powerful role of injury prevention strategies and explore practical steps that not only shield us from harm but also enable us to thrive in our athletic pursuits.

Understanding Injury Prevention

Injury prevention isn't just about avoiding harm; it's about nurturing the longevity of our athletic journey. The cumulative effects of training, coupled with the natural changes in our bodies, necessitate a strategic approach that combines mindfulness, preparation, and adaptive training.

Foundations of Injury Prevention: Tips and Strategies

- **Prioritize Warm-Up and Cool-Down**: Dedicate ample time to warming up your body before engaging in physical activity. Dynamic movements like leg swings, arm circles, and light aerobic exercises increase blood flow and prepare your muscles for action. After your workout, engage in static stretches to promote flexibility and ease muscle tension.

- **Listen to Your Body**: The wisdom of age extends to knowing when to push and when to pull back. Learn to differentiate between discomfort and pain. If an exercise or movement causes pain, modify it or seek professional advice.

- **Incorporate Functional Mobility Exercises**: Dynamic stretches that mimic the movements you'll be engaging in during your workout help improve joint range of motion and reduce the risk of injury.

- **Mindful Strength Training**: Strength training is a cornerstone of injury prevention. Focus on compound movements that engage multiple muscle groups, mirroring functional training principles. Gradually increase weights and repetitions to build strength progressively.

- **Flexibility and Balance Routines**: Regularly integrate yoga, Pilates, or dedicated flexibility training into your regimen. These practices enhance joint mobility, improve balance, and maintain overall body suppleness.

- **Footwear and Equipment**: Invest in appropriate footwear and sports gear that provide the necessary support and cushioning for your chosen activities. Ill-fitting or worn-out shoes can contribute to discomfort and injury.

- **Proper Nutrition and Hydration**: Nourish your body with a balanced diet rich in nutrients that support muscle recovery and bone health. Staying hydrated is equally important for maintaining tissue function and preventing cramps.

- **Rest and Recovery**: Adequate rest is crucial for preventing overuse injuries. Listen to your body's signals and ensure you allow sufficient time for recovery between intense workouts.

Sample Injury Prevention Routine: Body-Mind Harmony

Warm-Up:

- 5-7 minutes of light aerobic exercise (e.g., brisk walking, cycling).

- Dynamic stretches targeting major muscle groups, such as leg swings, arm circles, and trunk rotations.

Workout:

- **Squats with Overhead Reach**: Engage in controlled squats while reaching your arms overhead. This enhances lower body strength and shoulder mobility.

- **Glute Bridges**: Lie on your back with knees bent. Lift your hips off the ground while engaging your glutes and core. This exercise improves hip stability and lower back strength.

- **Plank with Shoulder Taps**: Assume a plank position and alternately tap your shoulders with your opposite hand. This challenges core stability and shoulder strength.

- **Hip Flexor Stretch**: Kneel on one knee, while the other leg is bent at a 90-degree angle. Gently push your hips forward to feel a stretch in the front of the hip. Hold for 20-30 seconds on each side.

Cool-Down: 5-10 minutes of static stretches, focusing on the major muscle groups engaged during the workout.

As we inscribe the chapter of injury prevention into our athletic journey, we equip ourselves with a shield of wisdom and prudence. By integrating these strategies into our training routines, we create a resilient foundation that enables us to savor the thrill of sports while preserving our bodies for the years ahead. Injury prevention isn't a solitary endeavor; it's a collective effort between our passion for movement and our commitment to nurturing the vessel that carries us forward.

Crafting Your Strategic Training Regimen

Aging gracefully and training strategically involves more than just physical exertion. It demands a holistic approach that encompasses nutrition, rest, and mindfulness. Adequate hydration supports tissue health, while a balanced diet nourishes our bodies for optimal performance. Sufficient rest allows for recovery and healing, and mindfulness techniques contribute to stress reduction, a factor often underestimated in injury prevention.

Your strategic training regimen must also be dynamic. Periodization, a method of cycling training intensity and volume, prevents plateaus and overtraining. Adaptability becomes our strength as we fine-tune our routines to accommodate the ebb and flow of life's demands.

Crafting Your Strategic Training Regimen: A Blueprint for Athletic Longevity

In the intricate mosaic of aging gracefully and training strategically, the design of your training regimen becomes the cornerstone. In this chapter, we unveil the art of crafting a strategic training plan—one that not only aligns with your goals but also adapts to the ebb and flow of life's demands. By delving into the nuances of periodization, rest, and adaptability, we unlock the secrets to sustaining a vibrant athletic journey that spans the years.

The Framework of Strategic Training

Strategic training extends beyond the confines of the gym; it encompasses nutrition, recovery, and mindfulness. This comprehensive approach respects the interplay between physical exertion and the body's need for rejuvenation.

Elements of a Strategic Training Regimen

- **Goal Clarity**: Define your objectives—whether it's enhancing strength, improving endurance, or maintaining overall health. Your training regimen should be tailored to meet these goals.

- **Periodization**: Instead of a linear approach, embrace the concept of periodization. This involves cycling through phases of varying intensity and volume. It prevents plateaus, reduces the risk of overtraining, and optimizes progress.

- **Balanced Nutrition**: Nourish your body with a diet rich in lean proteins, complex carbohydrates, healthy fats, and a variety of vitamins and minerals. These nutrients fuel your workouts and support recovery.

- **Hydration**: Maintain proper hydration before, during, and after your workouts. Water supports muscle function, joint lubrication, and overall bodily processes.

- **Rest and Recovery**: Dedicate time to rest and recovery. Adequate sleep allows your body to repair and rejuvenate, while active recovery days (e.g., gentle yoga, light walks) help prevent burnout.

- **Mindfulness Practices**: Incorporate mindfulness techniques such as meditation or deep breathing to manage stress. A calm mind complements a healthy body, contributing to injury prevention.

Sample Strategic Training Regimen: Holistic Harmony

Week 1-4: Strength and Foundation Building

- Focus on compound movements such as squats, deadlifts, and bench presses.

- Perform 3-4 sets of 8-10 repetitions at moderate weights.

- Incorporate dynamic stretches and functional mobility exercises before each session.

- Consume a balanced diet rich in lean proteins, whole grains, and vegetables.

- Aim for 7-8 hours of sleep per night.

Week 5-8: Endurance and Stamina Focus

- Introduce circuit training with minimal rest between exercises.

- Perform 3 sets of 12-15 repetitions at a lower weight range.

- Increase cardiovascular activities such as jogging, cycling, or swimming.

- Prioritize hydration before, during, and after workouts.

- Implement mindfulness practices, dedicating 5 minutes daily to meditation.

Week 9-12: Active Recovery and Flexibility

- Engage in light workouts focusing on flexibility, balance, and mobility.

- Incorporate yoga sessions or gentle Pilates routines.

- Emphasize hydration and consume anti-inflammatory foods like fruits and omega-3-rich sources.

- Dedicate time to self-care activities, such as foam rolling and hot baths.

- Maintain 8 hours of sleep for optimal recovery.

The architecture of your strategic training regimen is a canvas that marries ambition with prudence. By designing a regimen that adapts, rests, and renews, you create an enduring partnership between your goals and the resilient spirit that propels you forward. The chapters of your athletic journey are illuminated by the wisdom of periodization, the harmony of nutrition, and the serenity of mindfulness. As you step into each workout, you're not just sculpting your physique; you're nurturing a legacy of athleticism that gracefully defies the passage of time.

Embracing the Journey Ahead

As the chapter of your athletic journey unfolds, the tapestry of experiences weaves together with strategic training and injury prevention at its core. Through functional training, we sculpt our bodies not only to defy the effects of time but also to thrive in the face of challenges. This approach is a celebration of the wisdom we've gained, the determination that fuels us, and the passion that never wanes.

So let's lace up those shoes, roll out the yoga mat, and welcome each day with the enthusiasm of a seasoned athlete. For the road ahead is paved with both opportunities and obstacles, and our commitment to aging gracefully and training strategically will ensure that we traverse it with grace, strength, and joy.

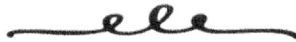

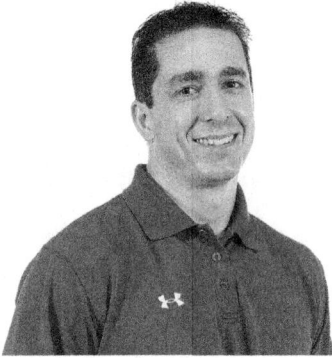

As a Registered Dietitian and Strength Coach with over 20 years of experience Jayson Hunter has seen just about every gimmick, fad diet and miracle pill you may have tried to lose inches fast. And while these "solutions" have worked for the short-term they've resulted in long-term disaster by wreaking havoc on your metabolism. Not only do you gain the weight back you lost, but you gain a whole lot more.

Something very interesting to note is that many of the hundreds of people that Jayson has helped had originally damaged their metabolism through starvation type diets they were using to lose weight for a special occasion. Some wanted to look great for their class reunion. Others wanted to fit into a bikini during their vacation.

The desire to makeover your body needs to be very strong to see results. And when are you going to have a greater desire than when you want to look great for a special day? Or for that vacation you've been wanting to take forever? There's no better time to discover the secrets to not only losing weight fast, but keeping weight off forever!

- Have you ever asked yourself or told yourself:

- Why can't I lose weight even when I don't eat hardly any calories?

- No matter what diet I try I can't seem to lose any weight

- I have a hard time sticking to diets

- Nothing looks good when I am on a diet

- What should I eat to lose weight?

 Or have you ever wished that you had someone that would tell you the correct way to lose weight. Where it would be successful and you wouldn't hate following the program or trying to lose weight.

.... You're in the RIGHT place!

As a Registered Dietitian and nationally known weight loss expert that has been featured on ABC, NBC, Fox, and CBS I am the one who **bridges the gap between what science does and what real world living does**.

Fully Alive Fitness Formula: The Fitness Blueprint For Middle-Age Career-Focused Individuals Looking For Life-Changing Results

By: Chris Baggett

In the bustling world of middle age, where career aspirations and family responsibilities often take center stage, the pursuit of personal well-being can easily fall by the wayside. Navigating the demands of a thriving career while maintaining a healthy lifestyle might seem like an unachievable challenge, but fear not. The Fully Alive Fitness Formula has been meticulously crafted to provide a comprehensive and sustainable fitness blueprint, specially tailored for individuals seeking to thrive in their careers while growing stronger Physically, Mentally, Spiritually, and Socially.

The Four Pillars of the Fully Alive Fitness Formula: The Heartbeat of Transformation:

- **Physical Transformation:** Ah, the pillar that often steals the limelight! Physical wellness is about more than just shedding a few pounds or lifting weights; it's the embodiment of energy, strength, and mobility. From workouts that challenge your body to nourishing meals that fuel your spirit, this pillar lays the foundation for a vibrant life. So, let's get those muscles moving and that heart pumping – after all, feeling strong physically sets the stage for feeling strong in all aspects of life.

- **Mental Empowerment**: Ever heard the phrase "mind over matter"? Well, it holds true here. Middle age can come with its fair share of mental hurdles, but the Mental Transformation pillar is your secret weapon. With mindful practices, stress-busting techniques, and a hearty dose of positivity, you'll be equipped to tackle challenges head-on. Remember, a healthy mind fuels a healthy body, and vice versa. So, let's flex those mental muscles and unleash our inner champions.

- **Spiritual Alignment:** No, we're not talking about levitating or summoning mystical creatures – though, that would be quite the workout! Spiritual Transformation is about finding that deeper connection within yourself. It's about nurturing your inner being, fostering gratitude, and seeking meaning beyond the surface. Whether you meditate, pray, or take solace in nature, this pillar reminds us that true well-being is an intricate tapestry woven with purpose.

- **Social Engagement:** Who said fitness had to be a solo gig? The Social Transformation pillar reminds us that we're all in this journey together. It's about building a supportive community that lifts you up and keeps you accountable. So, whether it's sharing laughs during workouts, teaming up for challenges, or simply enjoying a post-workout smoothie together, the bonds you create are as essential as the sweat you shed.

Conquering Physical Transformation: Efficient Workouts for Packed Schedules and Nutrition Tips to Fuel Your Success

In the whirlwind of middle age, time is a precious commodity. That's why we've tailored our approach to help you efficiently weave workouts into your packed schedule. We've curated workouts that pack a punch in a limited timeframe. Whether it's high-intensity interval training (HIIT) to rev up your metabolism or quick bodyweight circuits during lunch breaks, we're here to show you that quality workouts don't always demand hours in the gym.

Here are some samples workouts to suit various preferences and lifestyles:

HIIT Sample

High-Intensity Interval Training (HIIT) is your shortcut to an effective workout in a limited time. This HIIT session will leave you breathless and exhilarated. Perform each exercise for 40 seconds, followed by a 20-second rest. Complete the circuit 3 times for a total of 15 minutes.

- **Burpees:** The ultimate full-body move. Drop into a squat, kick your legs back into a plank, do a push-up, jump your feet back to your hands, and explode into a jump.

- **Squat Jumps:** Engage your legs and cardiovascular system with explosive squat jumps. Land softly and immediately go into the next jump.

- **High Knees:** Elevate your heart rate while engaging your core by bringing your knees up toward your chest as quickly as you can.

- **Mountain Climbers:** Elevate your heart rate with this dynamic exercise. Alternate bringing your knees toward your chest in a running motion.

- **Plank Jacks:** Start in a plank position, then jump your feet out to the sides and back in again. This works your core and elevates your heart rate.

Bodyweight Circuit Sample

Sometimes, all you need is your own body weight to get a killer workout. This circuit is designed to target various muscle groups while keeping things simple. Perform each exercise for 45 seconds, followed by a 15-second rest. Complete the circuit 4 times for a 20-minute workout.

- **Push-Ups (or Knee Push-Ups):** Strengthen your upper body with this classic move. Keep your core engaged and maintain a straight line from head to heels.

- **Squats:** Engage your legs and glutes by squatting down as if sitting in a chair. Keep your weight in your heels and chest lifted.

- **Plank:** Engage your core and maintain a straight line from head to heels. Focus on your breathing and keeping your body stable.

- **Glute Bridges:** Lie on your back, bend your knees, and lift your hips off the ground by squeezing your glutes.

- **Supermans:** Lie on your stomach and lift your arms, chest, and legs off the ground simultaneously. Engage your back muscles and hold for a second before lowering.

Sneaky Movement Integration ideas

Who said movement had to be confined to the gym? Sneak in activity throughout your day with these ideas that don't feel like traditional workouts:

- **Stair Climbing:** Opt for the stairs instead of the elevator. Challenge yourself to take a few extra flights each day.

- **Dance Breaks:** Put on your favorite music and have a spontaneous dance party in your living room. Dancing is a fantastic way to move and have fun.

- **Walking Meetings:** Instead of sitting in a conference room, take your meetings outdoors. Walk and talk to get your steps in while being productive.

- **Park Playtime:** Take your kids or pets to the park and engage in active play. Throw a frisbee, kick a soccer ball, or simply chase each other around.

- **Yard Work:** Gardening, mowing the lawn, and other yard chores are excellent ways to get moving without realizing you're exercising.

By integrating movement into your daily routine, you'll keep your body active and energized, all while enjoying life to the fullest. Remember, fitness isn't just about formal workouts – it's about embracing movement in all its forms!

Nutrition: The Fuel Igniting Success

Ah, nutrition – the secret sauce to igniting success. Just like a well-oiled machine, your body thrives when fueled with the right nutrients. At the heart of our nutrition philosophy lies the principle of balance – a symphony of whole foods that energize both body and mind.

- **Vibrant Veggies:** Picture your plate as a canvas waiting to be painted with a rainbow of colors. Load up on an assortment of veggies like leafy greens, vibrant peppers, crunchy carrots, and juicy tomatoes. These nutrient-packed powerhouses not only deliver essential vitamins and minerals but also add a burst of flavor and texture to your meals.

- **Protein Power:** Lean proteins are your muscles' best friends. Incorporate sources like chicken, turkey, fish, tofu, beans, and legumes to provide the building blocks your body needs for repair and growth. Protein also helps keep you feeling full and satisfied, which can curb those pesky snack cravings.

- **Whole Grains:** Swap refined grains for their whole counterparts. Think brown rice, quinoa, whole wheat bread, and oats. These complex carbs offer sustained energy and are rich in fiber, supporting digestion and helping you stay satiated.

- **Healthy Fats:** Don't shy away from fats – your brain and body love them. Opt for sources like avocados, nuts, seeds, and olive oil.

These healthy fats support brain function, provide energy, and contribute to that coveted glow in your skin.

- **Treats and Temptations:** Now, let's talk about treats. Yes, you heard that right – enjoying a slice of cake or a scoop of ice cream won't sabotage your efforts. It's all about finding the sweet spot between indulgence and nourishment. Remember, life is meant to be savored, and that includes the occasional indulgence.

- **Moderation Matters:** The key to success lies in moderation. Instead of adopting restrictive diets, embrace mindful eating. Listen to your body's hunger and fullness cues. Savor each bite, and eat with intention. By finding that balance between nourishing foods and occasional treats, you're cultivating a sustainable and enjoyable relationship with food.

- **Embracing Food Freedom:** To help you foster a healthy relationship with food, we encourage you to steer clear of labeling foods as "good" or "bad." Instead, categorize them as Green Light, Yellow Light, and Red Light foods. Think of your nutrition goals as a destination and your eating program as a journey. The more green lights you encounter, the quicker you progress towards your destination. Hitting some yellow or even red lights along the way doesn't mean you have to give up on reaching your destination.

As you navigate the grocery aisles and whip up delicious meals in your kitchen, remember that nutrition isn't just about numbers on a label. It's about the joy of cooking, the pleasure of savoring flavors, and the empowerment of fueling your body for all of life's adventures. With every wholesome choice you make, you're igniting a fire of success within – a fire that's fueled by vibrant veggies, protein power, wholesome grains, and the joy of living a life that's fully alive.

Mental Empowerment: Cultivating the Mental Landscape of Success

In the complexity of middle age, where career ambitions and family responsibilities intertwine, the journey to vibrant health is as much a mental expedition as a physical one. The power of your mindset cannot be overstated – it's the compass that guides your actions, shapes your habits, and ultimately determines your success. Let's delve into why mindset matters and explore samples of how to navigate and manage it throughout your middle ages.

The Power of Your Mindset

A positive mindset is a cornerstone of success, empowering you to overcome obstacles, embrace challenges, and celebrate victories. When you approach your fitness journey with a growth-oriented mindset, you're primed for learning, adaptation, and the resilience needed to thrive amidst life's demands.

Managing Your Mindset: Samples for Middle Ages

- **Cultivate Self-Compassion:** Middle age often comes with self-imposed expectations. Instead of dwelling on perceived shortcomings, practice self-compassion. Treat yourself with kindness and understanding, acknowledging that the journey has its ups and downs.

- **Embrace Change:** Middle age is a time of transition. Rather than fearing change, embrace it as an opportunity for growth. Adopt a mindset that welcomes new experiences, challenges, and the chance to learn from every twist in the path.

- **Set Realistic Goals:** Aspirations evolve, and that's okay. Set goals that are challenging yet achievable, creating a roadmap that excites and motivates you. Break larger goals into smaller milestones to celebrate along the way. remember you can't control the overall outcome, but what you can control is the behaviors that will help lead you to those outcomes

- **Focus on Progress, Not Perfection:** Perfection is a lofty goal, and striving for it can lead to frustration. Instead, celebrate the progress you make, no matter how small. Each step forward is a testament to your commitment and determination.

As you embark on this middle-age adventure, remember that your mindset is the captain of your ship. By cultivating a positive and growth-oriented mindset, you're equipping yourself to navigate the seas of change, embrace challenges, and celebrate every milestone along the way. The power to transform your middle ages into a chapter of growth, vitality, and fulfillment resides within your mindset. So, embark on this mental journey with open arms, an open heart, and an unwavering belief in your ability to thrive – because when your mindset aligns with your goals, anything is possible.

Finding Your Spiritual Alignment: A Journey Inward

Picture your inner self as a hidden garden, waiting for you to explore. Spiritual alignment is the key that unlocks this garden, inviting you to wander its pathways and tend to its blossoms. It's a journey that takes you beyond the busyness of life, into a space of stillness where you can hear the wisdom of your heart. It's about dedicating time to listen to your inner dialogue, understand your aspirations, and create a space for soul-searching.

Nurturing Your Inner Being

Just as you care for your physical body with workouts and nourishing foods, your inner being requires nurturing too. Spiritual transformation is like watering the roots of a plant – it revitalizes your sense of purpose, encourages self-compassion, and provides a sanctuary for your thoughts and emotions. Whether it's through meditation, journaling, or simply sitting in silence, these practices allow you to connect with your essence and tend to your emotional well-being.

Fostering Gratitude and Meaning

Ever noticed how a simple act of gratitude can light up your day? Spiritual alignment embraces gratitude as a beacon that guides you toward positivity. It's about acknowledging the blessings in your life, no matter how small, and infusing your days with appreciation. Beyond gratitude, it's also about seeking meaning in your experiences – finding purpose in both challenges and triumphs. When you live with intention and mindfulness, every moment becomes a piece of a greater puzzle.

Connecting with the Sacred

Spirituality isn't confined to sacred spaces; it's about recognizing the sacredness in everything. Whether it's a sunrise, a kind gesture, or the laughter of loved ones, there's a divinity woven into the fabric of life. This pillar encourages you to pause and acknowledge these moments, to find awe in the ordinary and to infuse your days with respect and love.

As you journey through the realm of Spiritual Alignment, remember that it's not about adhering to a set of rules or doctrines. It's about embracing a path that resonates with your heart, fostering a connection with your inner self, and recognizing the beauty and purpose that lie within every facet of your existence. Just as a tapestry is woven thread by thread, your spiritual alignment weaves a sense of depth, purpose, and awe into the canvas of your well-being. So embark on this inner exploration with an open heart, and let the magic of spiritual transformation guide you toward a life that's truly, unapologetically, and divinely fully alive.

Creating Social Engagement for Accountability and Support: Thriving Together in Community

In the tapestry of life, having a support system is like having a group of close friends – they're there to lift your spirits, celebrate your successes, and provide a sturdy foundation for your journey. Accountability, much like a reliable compass, guides you on this exhilarating adventure. And guess what? You're not embarking on this voyage solo – you're surrounded by fellow travelers, each playing their role to ensure your journey is marked by achievement and growth.

The Power of Accountability

Imagine having a fitness buddy who sends you a message, "Ready for that workout?" or a coach who checks in on your progress. Accountability isn't just about keeping tabs on your actions – it's a potent motivator that propels you forward, even when motivation falters. It's like having a North Star that consistently points you toward your goals, reminding you that every stride counts.

The Art of Supportive Communities

Being part of a community that shares your aspirations is like finding your stride in a group of runners. Online forums, workout classes, or even workout partners at the gym – these connections form the backdrop of your journey. Sharing challenges, victories, and even those moments of setback with like-minded individuals creates a bond that's as empowering as it is heartening.

Sharing Progress and Milestones

Imagine achieving a personal best in your workout, and you have an entire circle of supporters ready to celebrate with you. Sharing your progress and milestones with a community that genuinely cares transforms solitary accomplishments into collective triumphs. It's about receiving recognition for your commitment, understanding that your achievements inspire others to pursue their own goals.

The Motivating Effect of Encouragement

Ever had someone tell you, "You've got this!" when you're on the verge of giving up? That's the power of encouragement. In your fitness journey, encouragement serves as a gentle breeze at your back, giving you that extra nudge to conquer challenges. Whether it's a virtual thumbs-up, a heartfelt comment, or a virtual high-five after a challenging session, these small gestures wield significant influence.

The Collective Strength

Imagine an amalgamation of voices cheering you on – that's the collective strength of a supportive community. It's the reassurance that you're not alone in your struggles or achievements. It's the camaraderie that propels you forward, even on days when you're tempted to hit the snooze button. It's a network that helps you rise above obstacles and reminds you of your potential for greatness.

In the intricate fabric of your fitness journey, accountability and support are the threads that add resilience and vibrancy to your tapestry of well-being. As you surround yourself with individuals who uplift, inspire, and navigate the path with you, remember that together, you're crafting a portrait of success that's destined to inspire and echo through the chapters of your life. So, embrace the collective strength of creating social connections and let it guide you toward a future that's fully alive – a future where you flourish, not just as an individual, but as a part of a community that thrives.

Adapting To The Landscape Of Middle Age For Long Term Success

Change is the only constant, and your fitness journey is no exception. Just as the seasons transition, your body and life circumstances evolve, calling for a dynamic approach to wellness. Our bodies aren't static entities; they're harmonious compositions of change and growth. This is where the magic of adaptation comes into play. It's not about clinging to rigid routines, but about embracing the art of flexibility.

- **Embracing New Challenges:** Picture yourself as an explorer venturing into uncharted territory. As the years go by, you'll encounter new landscapes – and we're not just talking about physical landscapes. Your fitness journey extends beyond the gym floor; it's about exploring new activities, finding joy in different forms of movement, and challenging yourself in unexpected ways. Perhaps it's adding a dance class to your routine, trying out a new sport, or discovering the world of outdoor adventures. Embracing new challenges not only keeps your routine exciting but also ensures that you're continuously pushing your limits and evolving.

- **Adjusting to Changing Needs:** Your body is your best compass. As you navigate through middle age, it's crucial to listen to its cues. A workout routine that once felt invigorating might need adjustments as your body's needs change. Maybe you prioritize joint-friendly exercises or focus on maintaining flexibility. By staying attuned to your body's whispers, you can curate a routine that promotes longevity and well-being.

- **Prioritizing Self-Care:** In the hustle and bustle of middle age, self-care can often take a backseat. But adaptability means recognizing that your well-being is a priority. It's about creating space for rejuvenation, recovery, and mindfulness. Whether it's scheduling rest days, indulging in a spa day, or dedicating time to relaxation, self-care is the cornerstone of sustainability.

- **Consistency Through Change:** Amidst all this change, one element remains steadfast – your commitment to consistency. It's not about perfection, but about showing up for yourself, even when circumstances shift. Adaptation doesn't mean abandoning your journey; it means finding innovative ways to stay connected to your goals and nurturing your well-being.

So, as you cover the landscape of middle age, remember that adaptation is your trusty compass. It's not about resisting change, but about embracing it as an opportunity for growth and renewal. By evolving your routines, welcoming new challenges, and placing self-care at the forefront, you're setting yourself up for a fitness journey that's as enduring and vibrant as you are. In the symphony of change, you're the conductor – guiding the melody of your fitness journey with grace, enthusiasm, and an unwavering commitment to self-evolution.

Embracing the Fully Alive Fitness Formula: Thriving in Every Dimension

And there you have it, the Fully Alive Fitness Formula in all its dynamic glory! Your journey isn't just about physical transformation; it's about thriving in every dimension of your life. As you weave the threads of physical strength, mental clarity, spiritual connection, and social engagement, you'll create a tapestry of vibrant living. So, don't just follow this formula – embrace it with open arms, and let it guide you toward a life that's truly, unapologetically, and beautifully fully alive.

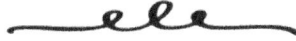

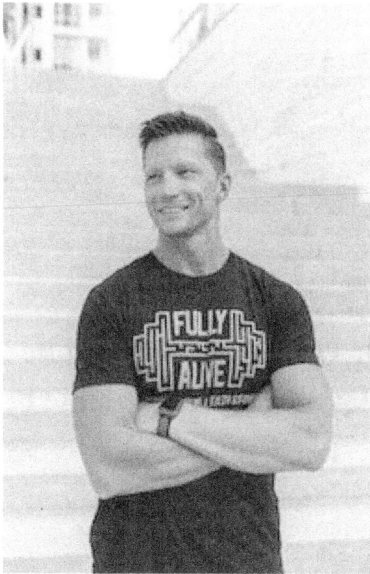

Meet Chris, the visionary force behind "Fully Alive Fitness Formula." With a remarkable journey spanning 14 prolific years in the fitness industry, Chris has sculpted his path as the founder of Fully Alive Personal Training and Health Studios. His unwavering commitment to transformation has empowered countless clients to navigate their wellness journey, fostering their evolution into the happiest and healthiest versions of themselves.

Throughout his dynamic career, Chris's adept guidance has left an indelible mark on diverse individuals seeking a holistic approach to fitness. With a genuine desire to uplift others, he intertwines his deep knowledge of training techniques with a contagious passion for life. Amidst kettlebells and cardio, you might even catch him sharing a witty dad joke or showcasing his legendary dance moves – because embracing health should be as enjoyable as it is rewarding.

Beyond the realms of fitness, Chris's personal story finds its harmony in his role as a devoted husband to his high school sweetheart, Leah, and a cherished father to Kailea and Chris Jr. Their presence illuminates the "why" behind Chris's lifelong mission: to radiate positivity and inspire transformative change. Rooted in this purpose, Chris envisions a world where his guidance not only helps individuals grow stronger physically but also propels them to cultivate mental resilience, spiritual well-being, and thriving social connections.

So step into the world illuminated by "Fully Alive Fitness Formula," where Chris's insights, honed through years of dedication, await. It's a testament to Chris's journey, a treasure chest of wisdom crafted through unwavering commitment.

Are you ready to embrace vitality in every fiber of your being? Chris' new book, **"Fully Alive Fitness Formula: The Fitness Blueprint for Middle-Age Career-Focused Individuals Looking for a Path to Life Changing Results,"** goes into much more details and provides the exact blueprint for living Fully Alive. You can grab his book for yourself at <u>https://keap.page/vzr301/fafitness.html</u>.

<u>www.Fullyalivept.com</u>

Phone (757) 301-9538

Stronger With Age: Cultivating Strength and Resilience After 40

By: Willie Ray

Embracing Strength and Resilience After 40: A Fitness Journey

This chapter is all about celebrating the fantastic forties and beyond, a time of life when wisdom and experience blend to create a unique tapestry of strength and resilience. It's time to kick off those worries about age and step into a world where you truly come into your own.

This detailed guide is your compass to navigating a holistic approach to fitness, encompassing both the physical and mental facets of wellness. So grab a cup of your favorite brew and let's dive into the beautiful journey of cultivating strength and resilience after 40.

The Marvelous Metamorphosis of Fitness

Consider your forties a period of metamorphosis, akin to a butterfly emerging from its chrysalis. Just as the caterpillar transforms into a resplendent creature, your forties usher in a metamorphic journey where strength and resilience intertwine to sculpt a masterpiece of wellness. The fitness goals you set in your twenties may have centered on aesthetics, while your thirties honed your balancing act between family, career, and self-care.

Now, in your forties, you're primed to embrace a holistic approach that not only invigorates your body but nurtures your mind and spirit.

This metamorphosis is a celebration of the beauty that comes with age—an age marked by wisdom, experience, and a deeper connection to self. As you delve into this chapter, remember that every step you take, every breath you draw, is a tribute to your remarkable journey.

The Resilient Workout Regimen

In your forties, your fitness regimen becomes an exquisite symphony of strength, designed to nurture your body's inherent resilience. Crafting a workout routine that resonates with this chapter means harmonizing different elements to create a balanced and robust fitness routine.

1. **Strength Training Symphony:** Think of strength training as the backbone of your fitness composition. Focus on full-body exercises that engage multiple muscle groups, such as squats, lunges, deadlifts, and overhead presses. By incorporating compound movements, you enhance muscle coordination and overall functional strength.

2. **Cardiovascular Cadence:** Your cardiovascular system is like the rhythm section of your fitness orchestra. Engage in activities that elevate your heart rate, such as brisk walking, jogging, swimming, or cycling. High-Intensity Interval Training (HIIT) can be a potent addition, alternating bursts of vigorous exercise with recovery periods to enhance cardiovascular fitness and fat burning.

3. **Flexibility Flourish:** Just as a symphony embraces various instruments, your fitness routine should include flexibility training. Practices like yoga or Pilates enhance joint mobility, reduce the risk of injury, and promote a

sense of tranquility. These sessions provide a harmonious counterbalance to more intense workouts.

Here's a sample workout that incorporates strength training, cardiovascular training, and flexibility exercises, tailored to cultivate resilience and vitality after 40:

Forties' Fitness Fusion Workout

Warm-Up (5-7 minutes):

Begin with light cardio, such as brisk walking, to elevate your heart rate and increase blood flow. Follow this with dynamic stretches like arm circles, leg swings, and hip rotations to prepare your body for the workout ahead.

Strength Training Circuit (3 rounds):

Perform each exercise for 12-15 reps, resting 45 seconds between exercises and 1-2 minutes between rounds.

1. **Goblet Squats**: Hold a dumbbell or kettlebell close to your chest. Lower into a squat, keeping your back straight and chest up. Push through your heels to stand back up.

2. **Push-Ups:** Perform classic push-ups or modify with knee push-ups. Keep your body in a straight line and engage your core as you lower and push back up.

3. **Bent-Over Rows:** Hold dumbbells with palms facing you, hinge at your hips, and slightly bend your knees. Pull the weights toward your hips, engaging your back muscles.

4. **Step-Ups:** Using a stable platform, step one foot onto it and drive through that heel to lift your body up. Step back down and switch legs.

5. **Plank with Shoulder Taps:** Start in a plank position on your forearms. Tap one hand to the opposite shoulder while maintaining a stable core.

Cardiovascular Training (Interval Training):

Choose your preferred form of cardio (running, cycling, jumping jacks) and perform intervals:

Work Phase: 30 seconds of intense effort (sprinting, cycling at a fast pace, or performing high knees).

Recovery Phase: 60 seconds of moderate-paced activity (walking, slow cycling, or jogging in place).

Repeat the work and recovery phases for a total of 5-7 rounds, gradually increasing the number of rounds as your fitness improves.

Flexibility and Cool Down (10-15 minutes):

Wrap up your workout with static stretches to enhance flexibility and promote relaxation:

1. **Hamstring Stretch:** Sit on the floor with one leg extended, the other bent. Reach for your toes on the extended leg, feeling the stretch in your hamstring.

2. **Quad Stretch:** Stand on one leg and bend your other knee, bringing your foot towards your glutes. Hold your foot with your hand and gently pull, feeling the stretch in your quadriceps.

3. **Child's Pose:** Kneel on the floor and sit back on your heels. Extend your arms in front of you and lower your chest towards the ground, feeling the stretch in your lower back and hips.

4. **Triceps Stretch:** Extend one arm overhead and bend your elbow, reaching down your back. Use your opposite hand to gently pull your bent elbow, feeling the stretch in your triceps.

Guidelines and Tips:

- Start with weights that challenge you but allow you to maintain proper form.

- Listen to your body and adjust the intensity based on your fitness level.

- Stay hydrated throughout the workout.

- Focus on controlled movements and proper breathing.

- Always cool down with stretching to improve flexibility and prevent muscle soreness.

Remember, this sample workout is just a starting point. Feel free to modify exercises, repetitions, and rest periods to suit your individual fitness level and preferences. The key is to embrace the fusion of strength, cardiovascular, and flexibility training to cultivate resilience and thrive in your forties and beyond.

Nutrition: The Fuel for Resilience

Like a symphony's orchestra requires a diverse range of instruments, your body thrives on a well-rounded nutritional palette. Fueling your body with the right nutrients is instrumental in nurturing your resilience and sustaining your fitness journey.

1. **Protein Partnerships:** In your forties, protein becomes your fitness concerto's leading soloist. Lean protein sources like chicken, turkey, fish, eggs, legumes, and plant-based proteins aid muscle repair and maintenance. Incorporating protein-rich meals after workouts supports recovery and encourages muscle growth.

2. **Mighty Micronutrients:** Your body's resilience is fortified by an ensemble of vitamins and minerals. Vibrantly colored fruits and vegetables are like the harmonious chords of a symphony, delivering a plethora of antioxidants that combat oxidative stress and promote overall well-being.

3. **Hydration Harmony:** Hydration is the rhythm that sustains your body's vitality. Adequate water intake is pivotal for energy levels, muscle function, and post-workout recovery. Aim to stay hydrated throughout the day, and consider beverages like herbal teas and infused water to enhance flavor.

Here's a sample meal plan that complements the theme of "Stronger With Age: Cultivating Strength and Resilience After 40." This meal plan focuses on providing nourishing, balanced meals that support your fitness goals, enhance resilience, and celebrate the wisdom that comes with age.

Day 1:

Breakfast:

- Scrambled eggs with spinach and tomatoes

- Whole-grain toast

- A side of mixed berries

Lunch:

- Grilled chicken salad with mixed greens, cucumbers, bell peppers, and a sprinkle of nuts and seeds

- Balsamic vinaigrette dressing

Snack:

- Greek yogurt with a drizzle of honey and a handful of almonds

Dinner:

- Baked salmon fillet with roasted sweet potatoes and steamed broccoli

- Quinoa pilaf with sautéed onions and garlic

Day 2:

Breakfast:

- Overnight oats made with rolled oats, almond milk, chia seeds, and topped with sliced bananas and walnuts

Lunch:

- Lentil soup with a side of whole-grain crackers

- Mixed fruit salad

Snack:

- Carrot and celery sticks with hummus

Dinner:

- Grilled turkey burger on a whole-grain bun with lettuce, tomato, and onion

- Baked zucchini fries

Day 3:

Breakfast:

- Whole-grain pancakes topped with Greek yogurt and fresh berries

Lunch:

- Quinoa salad with black beans, corn, diced bell peppers, and a lime-cilantro vinaigrette

Snack:

- Cottage cheese with sliced peaches

Dinner:

- Stir-fried tofu and vegetables with brown rice

- Steamed asparagus with lemon zest

Day 4:

Breakfast:

- Smoothie made with spinach, banana, almond milk, and a scoop of protein powder

Lunch:

- Grilled vegetable wrap with hummus in a whole-grain tortilla

- Side of mixed greens with olive oil and lemon dressing

Snack:

- Trail mix with nuts, seeds, and dried fruits

Dinner:

- Roasted chicken breast with quinoa and a side of sautéed Brussels sprouts

Day 5:

Breakfast:

- Avocado toast on whole-grain bread with a poached egg and a sprinkle of red pepper flakes

Lunch:

Mediterranean-style salad with chickpeas, cherry tomatoes, cucumber, red onion, feta cheese, olives, and a light vinaigrette

Snack:

- Sliced apple with almond butter

Dinner:

- Grilled fish tacos in whole-grain tortillas with cabbage slaw and a side of black beans

Meal Plan Guidelines:

- Prioritize lean protein sources like eggs, chicken, turkey, fish, tofu, and legumes to support muscle repair and maintenance.

- Incorporate a variety of colorful fruits and vegetables to provide essential vitamins, minerals, and antioxidants.

- Choose whole grains such as brown rice, quinoa, and whole-grain bread for sustained energy and fiber.

- Include healthy fats from sources like nuts, seeds, avocados, and olive oil to support overall health.

- Stay hydrated throughout the day by drinking water, herbal tea, or infused water.

- Opt for balanced meals that include a combination of protein, carbohydrates, and healthy fats to maintain energy levels and promote satiety.

Remember that this sample meal plan is just a starting point. Feel free to adjust portion sizes and ingredients to suit your dietary preferences and nutritional needs. The key is to nourish your body with wholesome foods that celebrate your forties and contribute to your strength, resilience, and overall well-being.

Mindful Movement and Self-Care Symphony

Just as a symphony conductor guides the orchestra, you lead the harmonious composition of your well-being. Mindful movement and self-care are the elegant notes that infuse your fitness journey with depth and vitality.

1. **Mindful Moments:** Incorporating mindfulness into your fitness routine transforms each workout into a meditative experience. Before and after exercise, take a few moments for deep breathing or meditation. These practices enhance your mind-body connection, fostering a sense of calm and awareness.

2. **Quality Rest:** Just as the pauses between musical notes create rhythm, rest is an essential rhythm in your fitness regimen. Prioritize quality sleep to support recovery and optimize the benefits of your workouts. Sleep is your body's natural way of restoring its symphony of systems.

3. **Restorative Rituals:** Self-care is the soothing melody that complements your fitness crescendo. Treat yourself to relaxing rituals like foam rolling, stretching, or a warm bath. These moments of rejuvenation alleviate muscular tension, reduce stress, and enhance overall well-being.

Embracing Challenges with Fortitude

Your forties are an era of empowerment, where every challenge becomes an opportunity for growth and triumph. Approach each workout with a mindset of fortitude and determination. Each exercise, each repetition, is a testament to your unwavering spirit.

Embrace the philosophy that you are not merely exercising; you are sculpting a future imbued with vitality and resilience. The strength you cultivate within the gym reverberates into every facet of your life, empowering you to face challenges with grace and tenacity.

In Conclusion: A Symphony of Strength and Resilience

As you navigate the symphonic journey of "Stronger With Age," envision your fitness routine as a composition that harmonizes strength, nutrition, mindfulness, and self-care. With every workout, you're composing a melody of resilience that resonates through time.

Your forties are a chapter of transformation, an anthem of strength that defies age and embraces experience. Celebrate your body's resilience, relish the journey, and savor the symphony of wellness that unfolds with each step, each lift, and each mindful breath.

So, let the rhythm of your forties propel you toward a future brimming with health, vitality, and an unwavering spirit of resilience. Your fitness journey is an ode to the magnificence of age—a testament to the symphony of strength and resilience that accompanies you through the remarkable chapter titled "Stronger With Age."

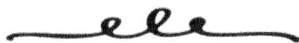

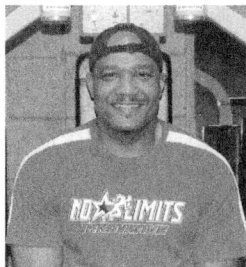

Willie B. Ray is a strength, nutrition, and body transformation coach in Lexington, Kentucky originally from Detroit, Michigan.

After Willie's professional career, he saw the lack of strength, mobility, conditioning and proprioception in most athletes as well as the average person. Willie realized that it was important to focus on movement patterns and not just the exercise. Exercise requires movement, but knowing how to move is essential. Willie uses numerous modalities to aid in the development of functional movement patterns. Willie has a unique background as a former all-natural pro competitive bodybuilder, powerlifter, collegiate/professional football athlete and a 2005 USA bobsledder. Now, his focus is on competing with himself to see how far he can progress his movement skills and apply that knowledge and experience to help people move, feel, and look better.

Willie is a firm believer that EVERYDAY IS AN OPPORTUNITY for Self Improvement. His methodology is to improve the body's ability to adapt to physical stress in all planes of the body due to the demands of physical fitness or everyday life movement patterns by incorporating the use of kettlebells, vintage dumbbells, vintage barbells, battle ropes, etc.

The objective is to have complete joint integrity and mobility, which will create more physical power causing the body to be more resilient and less prone to injuries helping you reach your objectives by breaking all limits and barriers. This essentially creates more efficiency in your workouts.

If you are able to train like an athlete, you'll be able to move pain free throughout all planes of the body and be more mobile and agile. This is Willie's No Limits-StrongStyle Kettlebell Methodology.

https://nolimitsinnovative.org

Super Parent's Guide to Healthier Living: Balancing Family and Wellness

By: Seth Scrimo

Once upon a time in a cozy suburban neighborhood, there lived a remarkable couple, Sarah and John, who were lovingly known as the "Super Parents" among their friends and neighbors. They had three energetic kids, a bustling household, and a calendar filled to the brim with school events, soccer practice, and playdates.

As Sarah and John went about their daily routines, they embraced their roles as parents with unmatched enthusiasm. They'd wake up early to make breakfast, pack nutritious lunches, and ensure the kids were ready for school. They juggled work, household chores, and extracurricular activities, all while being the best possible role models for their little ones.

Their secret, the one that made them the superheroes of their neighborhood, was their commitment to a healthier lifestyle. They understood that to care for their family, they needed to care for themselves as well. Balancing their children's needs with their own well-being was their mantra.

Sarah and John's journey to becoming Super Parents wasn't without its challenges, though. They realized that being a parent meant constantly walking a tightrope between family and personal health. There were moments of exhaustion, skipped workouts, and the temptation of fast food dinners.

But they didn't give up. Sarah and John educated themselves about the science of weight management, the power of nutrition, and the art of meal planning. They discovered the magic of mindful snacking, the efficiency of family fitness, and the importance of self-care.

Their story of transformation became a beacon of hope for their friends and neighbors. The Super Parents inspired others to embark on their own journeys to healthier living. Together, they formed a close-knit community dedicated to supporting one another.

Sarah and John's tale proves that being a super parent isn't just about what you do for your children; it's also about what you do for yourself. By embracing a healthier lifestyle, they became the superheroes their family deserved, setting an example that would shape their children's lives for years to come.

The Super Parent Lifestyle: Balancing Health and Parenthood

In the world of parenting, Sarah and John knew they were living the ultimate adventure. Their days were a whirlwind of responsibilities, from school runs to bedtime stories, and they wouldn't have it any other way. Yet, amid nurturing their children's growth, they realized that self-care was equally essential.

Balancing Act: Super Parents understood the art of balancing parenting and self-care. They recognized that becoming healthier not only improved their lives but also equipped their children with valuable life skills.

Cracking the Code: Understanding the Science of Weight Management

Before delving into practical strategies for healthier living, Sarah and John explored the science behind achieving and maintaining a healthy weight. They discovered that sustainable changes were the key.

Calorie Control: The foundation of their journey was learning to balance calorie intake with energy expenditure. This understanding set them on the path to better health.

Nutrition Hacks for Super Parents: Fueling Your Family's Success

Sarah and John understood that nutrition was at the core of their family's healthier lifestyle. They embraced various nutrition hacks and clever strategies to ensure their family received the best possible nourishment.

Balanced Eating: This hack wasn't about strict diets or deprivation but about enjoying a wide variety of nutritious foods that provided essential nutrients. They focused on including a rainbow of fruits and vegetables in every meal. Here are some breakfast, lunch, and dinner examples:

- **Breakfast:** *Rainbow Smoothie Bowl*: They started the day with a vibrant and nutritious breakfast. In a blender, they combined spinach, banana, mixed berries, and a splash of almond milk. The kids had fun decorating their bowls with colorful toppings like sliced strawberries, kiwi, and shredded coconut.

- **Lunch:** *Colorful Veggie Wraps*: Lunchtime became a chance to experiment with veggies. They prepared whole-grain wraps and filled them with hummus, sliced cucumbers, bell peppers, and grated carrots. The kids loved the crunch and the variety of colors.

- **Dinner:** *Baked Salmon with Veggie Medley*: For dinner, they often opted for baked salmon. They seasoned it with lemon, garlic, and dill, then roasted it in the oven. Alongside, they prepared a medley of roasted vegetables like broccoli, sweet potatoes, and cherry tomatoes. It was a visually appealing and nutritious meal.

Mastering Meal Planning: Strategies for Healthier Family Dining

The couple's meal planning expertise became a game-changer. They designed weekly meal plans that combined convenience with nutrition.

Plan Ahead: The strategy of creating meal plans saved them time, money, and the stress of daily cooking decisions. For instance, they set aside Sundays for meal prep, involving their kids in the process. Together, they prepared batches of healthy snacks like homemade granola bars and cut-up veggies with hummus, making nutritious choices easily accessible for everyone.

Sneaky Snack Attacks: Navigating Healthy Snacking for Parental Palates

Snacking was part of their family life, but Sarah and John made smart snack choices that benefited everyone.

Mindful Snacking: They learned how to enjoy snacks without mindless overindulgence. Teaching their children the art of choosing nutritious snacks that satisfy their cravings without compromising their health became a fun family activity. They even turned snack time into a mini cooking adventure by making baked sweet potato fries or yogurt parfaits with fresh berries.

Efficient Exercise: Maximizing Family Fitness

Sarah and John knew that maintaining a fitness routine as a family required a bit of creativity and efficiency. With busy schedules, they opted for quick and effective workouts that allowed them to stay active together.

Morning Family Circuit:

Warm-up: Start with a light jog or jumping jacks for 5 minutes to get everyone's heart rate up.

Circuit (3 rounds):

- Push-ups: 10 reps

- Bodyweight Squats: 15 reps

- Plank: Hold for 30 seconds

- Jumping Jacks: 20 reps

Cool-down: Finish with some gentle stretching, holding each stretch for 20 seconds.

Backyard Fun HIIT:

Warm-up: Play tag for 5 minutes, incorporating running, dodging, and laughter.

HIIT Set (4 rounds):

- Sprint to one end of the yard and back.

- 10 Burpees (modified for kids).

- 10 Mountain Climbers (each leg).

Cool-down: Lie on your backs and do some leg stretches followed by deep breathing exercises.

Dance Party Workout:

Warm-up: Put on your favorite upbeat music and dance freely for 10 minutes.

Dance Routine (2 rounds):

- High-energy dance moves for 2 songs (5 minutes each).

- Include moves like the twist, the moonwalk, and the running man.

Cool-down: Slow down the music and do some gentle stretches, holding each for 20 seconds.

These quick workouts were designed to be fun and engaging for the entire family. They not only kept everyone active but also provided an opportunity for bonding and creating lasting memories. Sarah and John found that by incorporating fitness into their daily routines, they set a positive example for their children and instilled a love for physical activity that would serve them well throughout their lives.

Prioritizing Self-Care: Strategies for Your Well-being

The couple realized that a healthier them meant a happier family. Prioritizing self-care became a necessity, not a luxury.

Stress Management: Managing stress allowed them to handle the demands of parenting with grace. They practiced stress-relief techniques like deep breathing and meditation together. Family movie nights with cozy blankets and homemade popcorn became a cherished tradition to unwind and connect.

Overcoming Obstacles: Staying Motivated for Your Family

Maintaining motivation was challenging, but they broke their health and fitness goals into achievable milestones.

Set Realistic Goals: They broke down their health and fitness goals into smaller, achievable milestones. For instance, they signed up for a local charity run as a family, turning training sessions into quality time together. Celebrating each success along the way, whether it was a faster mile or a new yoga pose, helped them stay motivated.

The Power of Sleep: Energizing for Super Parenting

Quality sleep was the unsung hero of their healthy living journey. They understood how sleep impacted both them and their children.

Sleep Habits: They created a sleep-friendly environment for the entire family. Adequate rest was essential for both physical and emotional well-being. They established bedtime routines, read bedtime stories, and ensured their children had consistent sleep schedules. This not only improved the kids' sleep but also gave Sarah and John much-needed downtime for relaxation and self-care.

Embracing Support Systems: Building a Healthier Family Together

On this journey to a healthier family, Sarah and John realized they didn't have to go it alone. Support systems, from family and friends to online communities, played a crucial role.

Online Communities: They connected with like-minded parents online, gaining inspiration, motivation, and shared experiences. These communities offered valuable insights and encouragement. For example, they discovered a family fitness challenge group that provided workout ideas and healthy recipe swaps.

In conclusion, Sarah and John's story demonstrates that being a super parent is about caring for your children and yourself. By embracing a healthier lifestyle, they became the superheroes their family deserved, setting an example that would shape their children's lives for years to come.

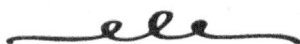

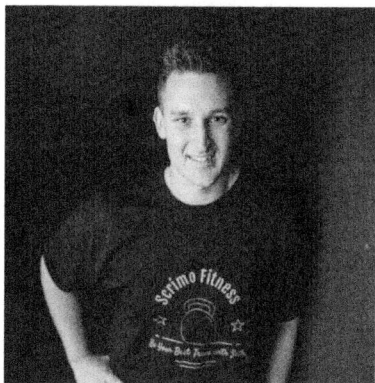

Seth Scrimo's experience in the health and fitness industry started with the United States Marine Corps in 2012. He enlisted in the Marine Corps Reserve while attending Kent State University. He knew that if he was going to become the best personal trainer he could be, he needed to learn from the best in the world.

Since graduating from Kent State University with a degree in Exercise Physiology in 2015 Seth has transitioned into becoming an American Council on Exercise Professional and holds unique

certifications such as Weight Loss Specialist, Diabetic Coaching and Fitness Nutrition Specialist. To better serve his clients before Covid-19 came to impact our lives, Seth went through a certification course to transition personal training programming to work online through the Online Training Academy in 2019.

Seth's niche of training is weight loss and body transformations. Seth has helped over 10,000 people change their lives and improve their health through systematic weight loss.

What Seth found is that most people over 30 who are struggling with their weight feel getting in great shape just isn't possible for them...

They no longer recognize themselves in the mirror, and they're tired of buying the next clothing size up. But they're too exhausted and overwhelmed taking care of everyone else, leaving little time or energy for their own self-care.

What they really want is to look and feel sexy in their favorite jeans, bathing suit, and even their birthday suit.

So they try every diet and exercise program under the sun with little-to-no results... and lots of frustration. It doesn't matter if they go keto or paleo, do HIIT or boot camps, take supplements, wear patches, or offer their own kids as a sacrifice to the weight loss gods... NOTHING WORKS!

Eventually, enough is enough, so they quit... again.

What they actually need is a weight loss program that meets them where they're at and fits into their busy schedule rather than trying to force themselves into an unrealistic, rigid program. Only then will they be able to achieve real results and finally feel confident in their bodies, take back control of their life, and be truly happy again.

Seth enjoys staying active outdoors. He runs long distance races for charity and early in the morning you can find him in the weight room working on building a stronger body. He enjoys reading and tries to listen to audio books throughout his day. Seth has a growing family and enjoys spending time with them outside of work. He volunteers at his church, where Seth helps sponsor their Youth Program to help mentor the young adults before they go out in life on their own.

You can connect with Seth at http://scrimofitness.com or scrimofitness@gmail.com

Seth's newest book, **"Slimming Secrets for Super Parents: Unlocking Weight Loss Success for Busy Moms and Dads"** goes into much more details and provides the exact blueprint for living the Super

Parent lifestyle you deserve. You can grab his book for yourself at **https://tinyurl.com/SlimmingSecretsForParents**.

Generation X: Navigating the Aches and Pains of Getting Older

By: Heath Herrera

In the grand tapestry of life, every generation weaves its own unique story. Generation X, known for its spirit of resilience, independence, and creativity, is now embarking on a new chapter - the journey of aging. With this passage of time comes an inevitable companion: the aches and pains that mark the transition into a more mature phase of life. This chapter delves into the nuanced experiences of Generation X as they navigate the physical changes that come with growing older, offering practical insights, friendly advice, and a compassionate perspective on embracing this evolving stage, while also highlighting the vital role of planning for longevity through health and exercise.

Embracing the Changes: A Natural Evolution

As members of Generation X step into their middle years and beyond, they may find themselves encountering a series of shifts in their physical well-being. The joints that once moved with youthful agility might now exhibit a hint of stiffness. Early mornings may be accompanied by the symphony of a few more cracks and pops than before. It's important to recognize that these changes are not indicators of decline, but rather the markers of a life well-lived. Each ache and pain tells a story, a testament to the adventures, challenges, and triumphs that have been woven into the fabric of one's existence.

A Lifelong Journey of Movement: Staying Active and Agile for Longevity

While the passage of time brings certain physical changes, it doesn't mean that Generation X must bid farewell to an active lifestyle. In fact, maintaining physical activity becomes even more vital in this stage of life. Regular exercise holds the key to preserving flexibility, enhancing muscle strength, and promoting cardiovascular health, all of which play a significant role in fostering longevity.

Engaging in activities such as walking, cycling, swimming, or practicing yoga can work wonders in supporting the body's vitality. These exercises not only help manage weight and reduce the risk of chronic conditions but also contribute to overall mental well-being, offering a sense of accomplishment and boosting mood.

Mind Over Matter: The Role of Mindfulness

As Generation X navigates the landscape of aging, they are equipped with a powerful tool to ease discomfort - the practice of mindfulness. Mindfulness involves being fully present in the moment, observing thoughts and sensations without judgment. This practice can serve as a potent antidote to stress, which can exacerbate physical tension.

Engaging in mindfulness techniques, such as meditation and deep breathing exercises, can contribute to a greater sense of calm and equilibrium. These practices not only alleviate stress but also create a space for individuals to develop a more compassionate relationship with their bodies, acknowledging and accepting the changes that come with age.

Building Resiliency Through Strength and Conditioning

In the timeless journey of aging, one thing remains abundantly clear: the body possesses a remarkable capacity for adaptation and renewal. For Generation X, embracing the aches and pains that come with getting older doesn't mean surrendering to them. Instead, it's an opportunity to harness the power of strength and conditioning to build resiliency and elevate the quality of life.

Strength Training: The Fountain of Youth

As the years gracefully advance, maintaining muscle mass becomes a pivotal element in the quest for a vibrant and resilient body. Engaging in regular strength training exercises can be likened to discovering a fountain of youth, as it contributes to numerous physical and mental benefits. By lifting weights, using resistance bands, or performing bodyweight exercises, Generation X can enhance muscle tone, bolster bone density, and fortify joints against the wear and tear of time.

Strength training goes beyond mere aesthetics – it directly impacts daily functionality. The ability to lift, carry, and move with confidence becomes an empowering asset that preserves independence and enables an active lifestyle. From lifting groceries to enjoying outdoor activities, the strength cultivated through focused workouts transforms the ordinary into the extraordinary.

Sample Full-Body Resiliency Workout

This sample workout is designed to enhance overall strength, improve muscular endurance, and promote balance and coordination. Incorporating a combination of lifting weights, using resistance bands, and performing bodyweight exercises, this routine offers a well-rounded approach to building resiliency for Generation X.

Warm-Up (5-7 minutes)

1. Jumping Jacks: 1 minute

2. Arm Circles: 1 minute (30 seconds forward, 30 seconds backward)

3. Leg Swings: 1 minute (30 seconds each leg)

4. Hip Rotations: 1 minute (30 seconds each direction)

5. Bodyweight Squats: 1 minute

Strength and Conditioning Circuit (3 rounds)

1. Lifting Weights: Dumbbell Squats

- Hold a pair of dumbbells by your sides at shoulder width.

- Stand with your feet shoulder-width apart.

- Lower into a squat by bending your knees and pushing your hips back.

- Keep your chest up and core engaged.

- Push through your heels to return to the starting position.

- Reps: 12-15

2. Resistance Bands: Bent-Over Rows

- Attach a resistance band to a sturdy anchor point.

- Hold the band handles with an overhand grip, palms facing your body.

- Hinge at your hips, keeping your back straight and core engaged.

- Pull the bands towards your hips, squeezing your shoulder blades together.

- Slowly release the tension to return to the starting position.

- Reps: 12-15

3. Bodyweight: Push-Ups

- Start in a high plank position with your hands slightly wider than shoulder-width apart.

- Lower your body towards the ground by bending your elbows, keeping your body in a straight line.

- Push through your palms to extend your arms and return to the starting position.

- Modify by performing push-ups on your knees if needed.

- Reps: 10-12

4. Lifting Weights: Dumbbell Lunges

- Hold a dumbbell in each hand by your sides.

- Step forward with one leg, lowering your back knee towards the ground.

- Keep your front knee aligned with your ankle and your chest upright.

- Push through your front heel to return to the starting position.

- Alternate legs for each rep.

- Reps: 12-15 per leg

5. Resistance Bands: Standing Shoulder Press

- Step onto the resistance band with both feet, holding the handles at shoulder height.

- Press the handles overhead, fully extending your arms.

- Lower the handles back to shoulder height with control.

- Reps: 12-15

6. Bodyweight: Plank with Leg Lifts

- Start in a high plank position, wrists under shoulders and body in a straight line.

- Lift one leg a few inches off the ground while maintaining plank position.

- Hold for a second or two, then lower the leg and alternate sides.

- Reps: 10-12 per leg

Cool Down (5-7 minutes)

1. Seated Hamstring Stretch: 1 minute per leg

2. Quadriceps Stretch: 1 minute per leg

3. Standing Calf Stretch: 1 minute per leg

4. Child's Pose: 1-2 minutes

5. Deep Breathing: 2-3 minutes

Remember to adjust the weights, resistance band tension, and repetitions to match your fitness level. Consult with a healthcare professional before beginning any new exercise program, especially if you have any pre-existing health conditions or concerns. This workout can be performed 2-3 times a week, allowing for adequate rest and recovery between sessions.

Conditioning: Breathing Life into Longevity

A well-conditioned body is a vessel of vitality, capable of embracing life's adventures with enthusiasm and endurance. Generation X can tap into the art of conditioning to enhance cardiovascular health, boost energy levels, and cultivate a robust respiratory system. Engaging in activities such as brisk walking, jogging, cycling, or swimming can elevate heart health, promote efficient oxygen utilization, and support optimal circulation.

Conditioning isn't solely about pushing physical boundaries; it also empowers the mind. The sense of accomplishment that accompanies reaching a new distance, completing a challenging workout, or conquering a steep incline carries over into daily life, fostering a can-do attitude and bolstering mental resilience.

Balancing Act: Enhancing Stability and Coordination

As the body matures, maintaining balance and coordination becomes increasingly important for preventing falls and injuries. Incorporating balance exercises into a fitness routine can work wonders in enhancing stability and sharpening reflexes. Activities like yoga, tai chi, and stability ball exercises challenge the body's equilibrium, promoting a strong core, improved posture, and confident movement.

Enhancing balance isn't solely about physical prowess; it also cultivates mental agility. The ability to navigate uneven terrain, step with confidence, and react swiftly to unexpected challenges translates to an increased sense of control and self-assurance in daily life.

Mind-Body Fusion: Strengthening Resilience on All Fronts

In the realm of strength and conditioning, the true magic lies in the interconnectedness of mind and body. Engaging in these exercises isn't just about sculpting the physical form; it's about fostering mental resilience, emotional well-being, and a heightened sense of self-awareness. The act of overcoming physical challenges through focused effort and determination becomes a metaphor for conquering life's hurdles with grace and tenacity.

Generation X can leverage the synergy between strength and conditioning to cultivate an unshakable sense of resilience. As they lift weights, traverse miles, and find balance within themselves, they forge a path toward longevity that extends far beyond the physical realm.

The Journey of Resilience

As Generation X embarks on the journey of aging, they hold within their grasp the tools to create a life marked by vitality, strength, and enduring resiliency. The pursuit of strength and conditioning isn't merely an endeavor to overcome the aches and pains that come with time; it's a bold declaration of agency and empowerment.

Through strength training, conditioning, and the cultivation of balance, Generation X can construct a body and mind that stand as testaments to their unwavering spirit. Each lift, each step, and each moment of balance achieved becomes a brick in the foundation of a life well-lived – a life that continues to flourish and inspire, a beacon of resilience for generations to come.

Fueling Wellness: The Nutritional Path

As the body matures, its nutritional needs also evolve. Generation X can support their well-being by adopting a diet rich in nutrients that promote joint health and overall vitality. Incorporating foods with anti-inflammatory properties, such as berries, leafy greens, nuts, and fatty fish, can help reduce inflammation and provide essential building blocks for maintaining optimal physical function.

Hydration, too, remains a cornerstone of well-being. Drinking an ample amount of water throughout the day aids in digestion, supports joint lubrication, and helps flush out toxins from the body. Additionally, consider incorporating supplements like omega-3 fatty acids or glucosamine, which have been shown to support joint health.

3-Day Anti-Inflammatory Meal Plan for Optimal Physical Function

Day 1:

Breakfast:

- Berry Smoothie Bowl

- Blend mixed berries (blueberries, strawberries, raspberries) with Greek yogurt, almond milk, and a handful of spinach.

- Top with sliced almonds, chia seeds, and a drizzle of honey.

Lunch:

- Grilled Chicken Salad

- Toss mixed greens, cherry tomatoes, cucumber, and bell peppers.

- Add grilled chicken breast, walnuts, and a vinaigrette dressing made with olive oil and balsamic vinegar.

Dinner:

- Baked Salmon

- Marinate salmon fillets in lemon juice, minced garlic, and olive oil.

- Bake and serve with steamed broccoli and quinoa.

Snack:

- Carrot Sticks with Hummus

Day 2:

Breakfast:

- Overnight Oats

- Combine rolled oats with almond milk, chia seeds, and a dash of cinnamon.

- Top with sliced banana, chopped walnuts, and a dollop of almond butter.

Lunch:

- Quinoa and Avocado Salad

- Mix cooked quinoa with diced avocado, chopped kale, pomegranate seeds, and a lemon-tahini dressing.

Dinner:

- Grilled Vegetable Stir-Fry

- Sauté a variety of colorful veggies (bell peppers, zucchini, mushrooms) in olive oil and garlic.

- Serve over brown rice with grilled tofu.

Snack:

- Handful of Mixed Nuts (such as almonds, walnuts, and pistachios)

Day 3:

Breakfast:

- Spinach and Mushroom Omelet

- Whisk eggs and pour into a skillet with sautéed spinach and mushrooms.

- Top with diced tomatoes and a sprinkle of feta cheese.

Lunch:

- Lentil and Kale Soup

- Prepare a hearty soup with lentils, kale, carrots, celery, and vegetable broth.

Dinner:

- Grilled Turkey Burger

- Make a lean turkey patty seasoned with herbs and spices.

- Serve in a whole-grain bun with lettuce, tomato, and a side of roasted sweet potatoes.

Snack:

- Greek Yogurt with Berries and a Drizzle of Honey

Tips:

- Stay hydrated throughout the day by drinking water, herbal teas, and infused water with cucumber and mint.

- Use olive oil as your primary cooking oil for its anti-inflammatory properties.

- Opt for whole grains like quinoa, brown rice, and whole wheat bread.

- Experiment with different herbs and spices to add flavor to your meals without relying on excessive salt.

Remember that individual nutritional needs vary, so it's important to consult with a healthcare professional or registered dietitian before making significant changes to your diet, especially if you have specific dietary restrictions or health conditions.

Connections and Community: Navigating Together

One of the hallmarks of Generation X is their ability to forge deep and lasting connections. These connections serve as a valuable resource as individuals traverse the landscape of aging. Sharing experiences, advice, and insights with peers who are also on this journey can provide a sense of camaraderie and understanding.

Forming or joining social groups centered around shared interests can provide a platform for exchanging tips on managing discomfort, discovering new wellness practices, and navigating the joys and challenges of aging. These interactions not only offer practical solutions but also remind individuals that they are not alone in their experiences.

Cultivating Holistic Wellness: Mind, Body, and Soul

As Generation X embraces the nuances of aging, it's important to recognize that well-being encompasses more than just physical health. Engaging in activities that nourish the mind, body, and soul holistically can contribute to a richer, more fulfilling life. Pursuing creative passions, whether it's painting, writing, or playing a musical instrument, fosters a sense of purpose and joy.

Quality sleep is another essential pillar of overall well-being. Establishing a consistent sleep routine, creating a calming bedtime ritual, and ensuring a comfortable sleep environment can promote restorative sleep and enhance the body's ability to heal and rejuvenate.

Planning for Longevity: Paving the Path to a Healthier Future

In the midst of embracing the present moment, Generation X can also harness the power of exercise and healthy living to lay the foundation for a longer, more vibrant future. Regular physical activity not only enhances current well-being but also has the potential to extend one's years of active, fulfilling life.

By making exercise a consistent part of their routine, Generation X can fortify their bodies against the effects of aging and reduce the risk of chronic conditions that can shorten life expectancy. Engaging in strength training, cardiovascular exercises, and balance-enhancing activities can contribute to maintaining mobility, independence, and a high quality of life well into the future.

In Conclusion: A Tapestry of Resilience and Longevity

In the grand tapestry of life, the journey of Generation X through the aches and pains of aging is a chapter of wisdom, strength, growth, and foresight. It's a testament to the resilience that has characterized this generation throughout their lives. Each ache and pain is a badge of honor, a mark of the experiences that have shaped them.

By staying active, embracing mindfulness, maintaining a balanced diet, nurturing connections, fostering holistic well-being, and planning for longevity through exercise and healthy living, Generation X can navigate this stage of life with grace and authenticity. As they continue to weave their story, the spirit of Generation X shines brighter than ever, an inspiration to all who follow in their footsteps, both now and in the years to come.

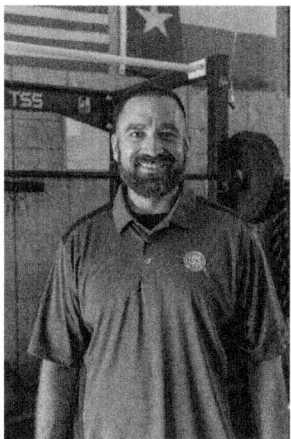

Heath Herrera, M.Ed., CSCS began his fitness career path by experiencing the absolute health and wellness that regular exercise and proper nutrition brought back to his own body. His own personal struggle and triumph gives Heath a superb ability to help nurture, motivate, and instill confidence in clients of all fitness levels and ages.

After topping out at 270lbs early in his life, Heath began a journey of weight loss, strength training, and conditioning that led to his eventual career path and what he uses to build physical longevity for his life. He has also gone through his struggles of depression and anxiety. Heath has taken the journey and continues to go down the path of cultivating a mind, body, and soul connection. Thanks to his personal struggles, as well as many years of professionally serving others, he has learned that every person is different and needs different motivations and methods to achieve his or her goals.

Heath began his coaching career as a Rehab Specialist helping injured workers get back to work quickly and safely. He helped individuals with sprained ankles, surgically repaired knees, carpal tunnel, strained backs, and many other injuries. Because of this experience, Heath is able to help individuals continue their treatment plan from their physician or physical therapist.

He then shifted to personalized coaching and group personal training (i.e. team training / boot camps), helping more people to get in front of the manageable and often times preventable injuries that keep them from enjoying life. With the transition from the rehab setting, Heath is able to combine the best of both worlds – working with individuals of all types to help them regain and retain their health, while helping to improve their quality of life.

Heath holds a Master of Education degree in Exercise Sports Science (2004) from Texas State University, San Marcos, TX and a bachelor's degree in Kinesiology (2002) from Angelo State University, San Angelo, TX. Heath is also a current member of the National Strength and Conditioning Association (NSCA) and is a Certified Strength and Conditioning Specialist (CSCS).

Email and/or website for contact info

Heath@HeathHerreraFitness.com

HeathHerreraFitness.com

Age-Defying Weight Loss: Thriving After 50

By: Peter Vasilis

Life after 50 is a remarkable period filled with opportunities for personal growth, adventure, and renewed vitality. Yet, for many, it can also be a time when maintaining a healthy weight becomes a bit more challenging. In this comprehensive guide, we will explore a range of simple, sensible, and effective weight loss solutions tailored specifically for adults over 50. Let's embark on this exciting journey to not only shed pounds but also enhance your overall well-being.

Understanding the Challenge

Before diving into the solutions, it's essential to understand the unique challenges that adults over 50 face when it comes to weight management. Several factors come into play, including:

- **Slower Metabolism**: With age, our metabolism tends to slow down. This means that the body burns calories less efficiently than it did in younger years.

- **Hormonal Changes**: Fluctuations in hormone levels, particularly during menopause for women, can affect weight distribution and make weight loss more challenging.

- **Muscle Loss:** As we age, we naturally lose muscle mass, which can further slow down metabolism and reduce calorie burn.

- **Lifestyle Changes**: Retirement, empty nesting, and changes in daily routines can lead to less physical activity and, sometimes, less attention to healthy eating habits.

Understanding these challenges will help you approach weight loss with realistic expectations and a tailored strategy.

Crafting Your Age-Defying Weight Loss Plan

1. Embrace a Balanced Diet

Nutrition remains a cornerstone of effective weight management at any age. Here's how to create a balanced, age-defying diet:

- **Portion Control**: Pay close attention to portion sizes. Using smaller plates can help you control portion sizes while still enjoying your favorite foods.

- **Nutrient Density**: Prioritize nutrient-dense foods such as fruits, vegetables, lean proteins, whole grains, and healthy fats. These foods provide essential nutrients while helping you feel full and satisfied.

- **Meal Timing**: Consider eating smaller, more frequent meals to maintain steady energy levels and curb cravings.

- **Hydration:** Ensure you drink plenty of water throughout the day. Sometimes, thirst is mistaken for hunger, leading to unnecessary snacking.

Here's a sample 3-day weight loss meal plan for adults over 50. This plan emphasizes nutrient-dense, balanced meals to help you achieve your weight loss goals while ensuring you get essential nutrients for overall health.

Day 1:

Breakfast:

- Scrambled eggs with spinach and tomatoes

- Whole-grain toast

- A small serving of mixed berries

Lunch:

- Grilled chicken breast salad with mixed greens, cucumbers, cherry tomatoes, and a vinaigrette dressing

- A serving of quinoa or brown rice

Snack:

- Greek yogurt with a drizzle of honey and a sprinkle of almonds

Dinner:

- Baked salmon with lemon and herbs

- Steamed broccoli

- Mashed sweet potatoes

Snack (if needed):

- Sliced bell peppers with hummus

Day 2:

Breakfast:

- Oatmeal made with old-fashioned oats, topped with sliced bananas and a dash of cinnamon

- A handful of mixed nuts (almonds, walnuts, and pistachios)

Lunch:

- Turkey and avocado whole-grain wrap with lettuce and tomatoes

- A side of carrot and celery sticks with a yogurt-based dip

Snack:

- A small apple with a tablespoon of almond butter

Dinner:

- Grilled shrimp and vegetable kebabs with a side of quinoa

- Steamed asparagus

Snack (if needed):

- Low-fat cottage cheese with pineapple chunks

Day 3:

Breakfast:

- Greek yogurt parfait with layers of yogurt, fresh berries, and granola

- A boiled egg on the side

Lunch:

- Lentil and vegetable soup

- A mixed green salad with balsamic vinaigrette

- Whole-grain crackers

Snack:

- Sliced cucumber and cherry tomatoes with a sprinkle of feta cheese

Dinner:

- Baked chicken breast with rosemary and garlic

- Roasted Brussels sprouts

- Quinoa pilaf with mixed vegetables

- Snack (if needed):

- Sliced pear with a handful of walnuts

Remember to adjust portion sizes according to your individual calorie needs and activity level. Staying hydrated by drinking plenty of water throughout the day is also essential for successful weight loss. Additionally, try to incorporate regular physical activity into your routine to complement your meal plan for even better results. Consulting a healthcare professional or registered dietitian for personalized guidance is always a good idea, especially if you have specific dietary restrictions or health concerns.

2. Stay Active

Regular physical activity remains crucial for weight management and overall health. Here's a detailed plan for incorporating exercise into your daily life:

- **Aerobic Exercise**: Aim for at least 150 minutes of moderate-intensity aerobic activity per week. Activities like brisk walking, swimming/aquatic exercise, and cycling are excellent choices. Break this down into 30-minute sessions, five days a week.

- **Strength Training**: As you age, maintaining muscle becomes even more critical. Incorporate strength training exercises into your routine at least two days a week. These exercises can include weightlifting, resistance bands, or bodyweight exercises.

- **Flexibility and Balance**: Include exercises that improve flexibility and balance. Yoga, Tai Chi, and stretching routines can help prevent injuries and maintain mobility.

3. Prioritize Strength Training

As mentioned, strength training is vital for preserving muscle mass and boosting metabolism. Here's a more detailed look at how to make it work for you:

- **Start Gradually**: If you're new to strength training, begin with light weights or resistance bands to avoid injury. Consult a fitness professional if needed.

- **Full-Body Workouts**: Focus on full-body exercises to engage multiple muscle groups simultaneously. Squats, lunges, push-ups, and planks are excellent choices.

- **Progressive Overload**: Gradually increase the weight or resistance over time to continue challenging your muscles.

- **Recovery**: Allow your muscles to recover between strength training sessions. This is when they grow stronger.

Here's a sample workout plan tailored for adults over 50 that starts gradually, offers full-body workouts, incorporates progressive overload, and emphasizes proper recovery. Remember to consult with a fitness professional before starting any new exercise program, especially if you have any existing medical conditions or concerns.

Week 1: Building a Foundation

Day 1 - Full Body Strength Workout:

- Bodyweight squats: 2 sets of 10 repetitions

- Wall push-ups (easier on joints than traditional push-ups): 2 sets of 8-10 repetitions

- Planks (start with a 20-30 second hold): 2 sets

- Rest between sets: 1-2 minutes

Day 2 - Active Rest:

- A 30-minute walk or gentle yoga/stretching routine

Day 3 - Cardio and Balance:

- Stationary cycling or brisk walking: 20-30 minutes

- Standing on one leg for balance (hold on to a sturdy support if needed): 2 sets of 30 seconds per leg

- Rest between sets: 1-2 minutes

Day 4 - Active Rest:

- A 30-minute walk or gentle yoga/stretching routine

Day 5 - Full Body Strength Workout (same as Day 1):

- Bodyweight squats: 2 sets of 10 repetitions

- Wall push-ups: 2 sets of 8-10 repetitions

- Planks: 2 sets

- Rest between sets: 1-2 minutes

Day 6 - Active Rest:

- A 30-minute walk or gentle yoga/stretching routine

Day 7 - Rest Day:

- Allow your body to recover

Week 2: Adding Complexity

Day 1 - Full Body Strength Workout:

- Bodyweight squats: 3 sets of 10 repetitions

- Wall push-ups: 3 sets of 8-10 repetitions

- Planks (try to increase hold time by 5-10 seconds): 2 sets

- Rest between sets: 1-2 minutes

Day 2 - Active Rest:

- A 30-minute walk or gentle yoga/stretching routine

Day 3 - Cardio and Balance:

- Stationary cycling or brisk walking: 20-30 minutes

- Standing on one leg for balance (try to increase hold time): 2 sets per leg

- Rest between sets: 1-2 minutes

Day 4 - Active Rest:

- A 30-minute walk or gentle yoga/stretching routine

Day 5 - Full Body Strength Workout (same as Day 1):

- Bodyweight squats: 3 sets of 10 repetitions

- Wall push-ups: 3 sets of 8-10 repetitions

- Planks: 2 sets (increase hold time)

- Rest between sets: 1-2 minutes

Day 6 - Active Rest:

- A 30-minute walk or gentle yoga/stretching routine

Day 7 - Rest Day:

- Allow your body to recover

Week 3 and Beyond: Progression

Continue to gradually increase the intensity, repetitions, and duration of your workouts as your fitness improves. Consider incorporating light dumbbells or resistance bands for added resistance in strength exercises. Listen to your body and adjust the plan as needed to ensure proper recovery and minimize the risk of injury. Always prioritize proper form over lifting heavier weights.

Remember, consistency is key to seeing progress. Incorporating full-body strength, cardiovascular, and balance exercises in a progressive manner will help you maintain and improve your overall fitness as an active-aging adult over 50.

4. Get Quality Sleep

Quality sleep is often overlooked, but plays a significant role in weight management. Here's how to optimize your sleep patterns:

- **Consistent Schedule**: Go to bed and wake up at the same time each day, even on weekends.

- **Create a Relaxing Bedtime Routine**: Wind down before sleep with activities like reading, gentle stretching, or relaxation exercises.

- **Sleep Environment**: Ensure your sleep environment is conducive to rest. Keep your bedroom dark, quiet, and at a comfortable temperature.

5. Manage Stress

Stress can significantly contribute to weight gain, especially in older adults. Here are some detailed strategies to manage stress effectively:

- Mindfulness Meditation: Consider practicing mindfulness meditation for as little as 10 minutes a day to reduce stress levels.

- Deep Breathing Exercises: Engage in deep breathing exercises when you feel stressed or anxious. Deep breaths can help calm the nervous system.

- **Engage in Hobbies**: Pursue hobbies or activities you enjoy to reduce stress and boost your mood.

- **Social Connections**: Maintain strong social connections with friends and family. Talking with loved ones can provide emotional support during stressful times.

6. Seek Support

Weight loss can be challenging, but you don't have to go it alone. Consider these supportive measures:

- **Join a Weight Loss Group**: Joining a weight loss group or support community can provide motivation, accountability, and a sense of belonging.

- **Hire a Fitness Professional**: A fitness professional can create a customized exercise plan and help you stay on track.

- **Consult a Nutrition Coach**: A nutrition coach can provide tailored nutrition guidance based on your specific needs and goals.

- **Involve Your Loved Ones**: Engage your family and friends in your weight loss journey. Their support can make a significant difference.

7. Monitor Progress

Keeping track of your progress is crucial for staying on course. Here's how to do it effectively:

- **Food Journal**: Maintain a detailed food journal to record your meals, snacks, and beverages. This can help you identify patterns and areas for improvement.

- **Exercise Log**: Log your workouts, including the type of exercise, duration, and intensity. This can help you monitor your progress and make adjustments as needed.

- **Weight and Measurements**: Regularly measure your weight and body measurements to track changes over time. Remember that fluctuations are normal and not always indicative of progress.

- **Mobile Apps and Technology**: Consider using mobile apps or wearable fitness trackers to streamline tracking and receive real-time feedback.

8. Be Patient and Persistent

Weight loss is a journey that takes time, especially for older adults. Be patient with yourself and stay persistent, even if progress is slow. Keep these detailed tips in mind:

- **Celebrate Small Wins**: Acknowledge and celebrate your achievements, no matter how small. Every step forward is a step in the right direction.

- **Set Realistic Goals**: Set achievable, realistic goals that align with your age, health, and lifestyle. Avoid setting yourself up for disappointment with overly ambitious targets.

- **Stay Consistent**: Consistency is key. Even on challenging days, do your best to maintain your healthy habits.

- **Seek Professional Guidance:** If you're struggling to achieve your goals or have specific health concerns, don't hesitate to consult a healthcare professional, such as a doctor or registered dietitian.

Conclusion

Age-defying weight loss is entirely achievable for adults over 50. By crafting a balanced diet, staying active, prioritizing strength training, getting quality sleep, managing stress, seeking support, monitoring progress, and maintaining patience and persistence, you can not only shed unwanted pounds but also enhance your overall quality of life.

Remember, it's never too late to embark on a journey to a healthier and happier you. The years after 50 are a time to savor life's moments, explore new interests, and enjoy the fruits of your labor. Your health and well-being are valuable assets that deserve your attention and care.

As you navigate the path to age-defying weight loss, keep in mind that the journey is as important as the destination. Embrace the daily victories, relish the newfound energy, and revel in the improved sense of self that accompanies your efforts. Share your journey with friends and loved ones and let them inspire you in return.

In the end, age is just a number, and your body has incredible resilience. With determination and these proven strategies, you can rewrite the script on aging, redefining what it means to thrive in your 50s and beyond. So, take that first step today and embark on a lifelong adventure towards a healthier, more vibrant you. The best chapters of your life are still waiting to be written – start writing them now.

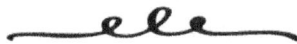

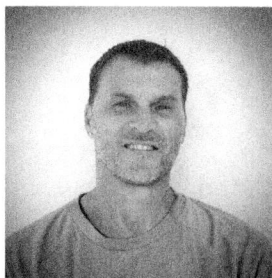

Peter Vasilis is a dedicated advocate for health and wellness, with a profound mission to empower individuals over 50 lead healthier, more fulfilling lives. With an extensive background in fitness and nutrition, he has become a trusted guide for those seeking sensible weight loss and an enhanced overall well-being through positive lifestyle changes.

As a seasoned fitness expert, Peter understands the unique challenges that individuals face as they age. With unwavering commitment, he has made it his life's mission to help men and women over 50 achieve their health and fitness goals. Through his holistic approach, he combines a sensible approach to exercise and presents the science of nutrition in simple terms to create transformative experiences for his clients.

As an "Active Ager" himself, Peter understands the physical and emotional aspects of aging. He recognizes that achieving sensible weight loss isn't just about shedding pounds; it's about reclaiming vitality and regaining confidence in our abilities & our bodies.

When he's not guiding clients toward their fitness goals, Peter enjoys staying active himself. He's an avid hiker, a sports enthusiast, and a lifelong learner who continues to stay updated with the latest advancements in fitness and nutrition.

With a firm belief in the power of education, Peter ensures that his clients are well-informed about the principles of healthy living. He guides them through the intricacies of nutrition and exercise, empowering them to make informed choices and sustain their progress for a lifetime. Through his unwavering dedication and expertise, he continues to make a profound impact, showing that it's never too late to embark on a journey toward a healthier, happier you.

Peter Vasilis is the owner of SlenderSense Weight Loss & Wellness Solutions, a company dedicated to empowering men and women over 50, achieve their weight loss goals simply & sensibly while improving their overall well-being and helping them achieve a lifetime of vitality and fulfillment. SlenderSense is a haven for those seeking sustainable lifestyle changes and positive transformations.

To discover how SlenderSense can help you achieve your weight loss & wellness goals and improve your overall lifestyle visit www.SlenderSense.com or email support@slendersense.com

Sole Mates: Your Feet's Journey from Neglect to Empowerment

By: Julie Anne McGready

Most days, we stick our feet into shoes and go about our business without giving them a second thought. It's easy to forget the incredible complexity and importance of our feet until they start to hurt, and generally by that time, there's often a real issue going on. Have you ever stopped to wonder about the marvels of your feet, or how they affect your overall health and fitness, especially as you've reached the age of 50 or beyond? Let's explore this together.

The Marvelous Machinery of Your Feet

Your feet are an engineering marvel, but we often take them for granted. Considering that each foot is composed of a staggering 26 bones, 33 joints, and over 100 muscles, tendons, and ligaments, they're responsible for much more than just carrying you from point A to point B. There are 206 bones in the adult human body, with feet making up approximately 25% of the total number. These bones work together to provide support, balance, and mobility, making the feet a critical part of our overall skeletal system. The muscles in your feet play a crucial role in maintaining balance, stability, and supporting the body's weight during activities like standing, walking, and running.

Bones of the Feet

- **Tarsal Bones (7):** These are the bones that make up the ankle and heel.

- **Metatarsal Bones (5):** The long bones connecting the tarsal bones to the toes.

- **Phalanges (14):** The toe bones, with three in each toe except for the big toe, which has two.

Muscles of the Feet

Within this complex structure, there are two primary groups of muscles: intrinsic and extrinsic. Intrinsic muscles are entirely within the foot, controlling its intricate movements. Extrinsic muscles, originating in the leg, have tendons that pass through the foot to help control its movements.

The Purpose of Your Feet

Ever considered why you have feet in the first place? Your feet serve two fundamental purposes:

1. **Adaptation to Terrain:** The forward foot's primary function is to conform to the surface you're walking on. It sends sensory signals up your body, allowing it to react and maintain balance.

2. **Propulsion:** The rear foot forms a rigid lever for push-off, propelling your body forward as you move.

Dynamic Foot Function During Gait and Movement

Your feet should have an equal distribution of mobility (for adaptation) and stability (for push off) to adapt during various movements. Understanding this dynamic function is key to appreciating their role in your health and fitness:

- During the gait cycle, your forward foot's toes are designed to widen and lengthen as they contact the ground. This spreads your weight evenly and maximizes stability.

- When you squat, sit, lunge, or exercise, your feet should also adapt by widening and lengthening, providing a broader base of support and enhancing balance.

Enhancing Leg Muscle Engagement with the Foot Tripod Position

Working your feet in a tripod position during exercise can significantly enhance leg muscle engagement, including the glutes, in a more natural and effective way. The foot tripod position involves distributing your body weight evenly across three key points on your foot:

1. The base of your big toe.

2. The base of your little toe.

3. The center of your heel.

By consciously activating and maintaining this tripod position during exercises such as squats, lunges, or even standing, you can:

- **Activate the Glutes:** The tripod position encourages the activation of your glute muscles, which are crucial for hip stability and overall lower body strength. When your feet are correctly aligned, your glutes can work in harmony with other leg muscles, promoting balanced muscle development.

- **Strengthen the Entire Leg:** This approach allows for a more even distribution of force through the entire leg, from the feet up to the hips. It reduces the risk of overloading one area, such as the knees, while underutilizing others.

- **Improve Balance and Stability:** The foot tripod position enhances your balance and stability by creating a solid foundation. This is particularly important as we age, as it reduces the risk of falls and related injuries.

- **Reduce Strain and Injury:** When your feet are aligned in the tripod position, there's less likelihood of undue strain on ligaments, tendons, and joints, reducing the risk of injuries over time.

Incorporating this mindful approach to foot positioning during your workouts can lead to more effective leg muscle engagement, better overall balance, and a reduced risk of injuries. Your feet play a pivotal role in this process, serving as the foundation upon which your leg muscles can build better strength and stability.

Proper Footwear

The choice of footwear plays a crucial role in foot health as well, and it's essential to consider the ramifications of certain types of shoes:

- **Tight Shoes (such as Dress Shoes):** Many of us have worn dress shoes that look sleek but offer little room for the natural expansion of our feet during the day. Over time, this can lead to issues like bunions, hammer toes, and ingrown toenails. To combat this, select dress shoes that allow adequate toe room and consider opting for wider widths if available.

- **High Heels:** While high heels can be fashionable, they can also be detrimental to your feet. They force your body into an unnatural position, pushing your weight forward onto the balls of your feet. This can lead to metatarsalgia (pain in the ball of the foot), plantar fasciitis, formation of bunions, calf tightness and hip and/or back issues. Limit high heel use, opt for lower heels when possible, and prioritize comfort and support.

- **The Unshod Foot:** The unshod (bare) foot is naturally wide and designed to provide maximum stability and proprioception (awareness of body position). When we encase our feet in shoes all the time, especially those with narrow toe boxes, it restricts the natural expansion of our feet. Spending some time barefoot can be beneficial for foot health, but be mindful of your environment to avoid injury.

Common Foot Issues in the 50+ Population

As we age, our feet face unique challenges, and understanding these challenges is really important for maintaining foot health:

1. **Arthritis:** Years of wear and tear can lead to foot arthritis, causing stiffness and pain. Arthritis in the feet often affects the joints of the toes, leading to discomfort and reduced mobility.

2. **Reduced Mobility:** Aging may bring decreased foot flexibility and range of motion. Conditions like tendonitis, which can cause inflammation and pain in the Achilles tendon, may become more common.

3. **Balance Concerns:** A natural decline in balance can increase the risk of falls and injuries. Conditions like peripheral neuropathy, which can cause numbness and tingling in the feet, may exacerbate these balance issues.

4. **Bunions:** Bunions are a common foot issue, especially among older adults. They are characterized by a bony bump at the base of the big toe, often causing discomfort and affecting foot alignment.

5. **Hammer Toes:** Hammer toes occur when the middle or end joint of the toe becomes bent, causing the toe to curl downward or buckle up. This condition can be painful and may affect the choice of footwear.

6. **Plantar Fasciitis:** Plantar fasciitis is a painful condition involving inflammation of the tissue that runs across the bottom of the foot. It can be especially problematic in the morning or after prolonged

periods of rest.

But Wait . . . There's Hope! Caring for Your Feet

Now, let's consider how you can care for your feet, especially considering these common issues:

1. **Foot Exercises:** Incorporate exercises to strengthen foot muscles and improve flexibility. One effective exercise involves sitting in a good position, on your sits bones, with your knees at 90 degrees and your ankles under your knees. In this position, focus on the foot tripod position - ensuring equal weight distribution between the base of your toes and the center of your heels. Gently lift your toes just off the floor while maintaining the tripod position, then lengthen them without twisting or gripping. Hold this lengthened position for 3 seconds, relax, and repeat. Aim for 3 sets of 5 repetitions. Doing this exercise in front of a mirror can be beneficial to ensure proper form.

2. **Proper Footwear:** Shoes mean something different for everyone, it's not a one shoe fits all. Generally speaking, they should be flexible with wider toe boxes that promote good foot alignment. If you have bunions or hammer toes, seek out shoes with ample toe box space.

3. **Regular Check-ups:** Visit a podiatrist for periodic foot check-ups, especially if you experience pain or discomfort. Early intervention can prevent minor issues from becoming major problems.

4. **Foot Massage and Stretching:** Regular massages and stretches can relieve tension and promote blood circulation. Consider toe stretches, ankle circles, and calf stretches to maintain flexibility.

5. **Orthotic Inserts:** In some cases, individuals may benefit from custom orthotic inserts designed to support and optimize foot function. These inserts should be considered after a thorough evaluation by a healthcare professional.

6. **There Is Hope for Your Feet:** No matter what challenges your feet may be facing, there is hope for improvement. Through a combination of exercises, proper footwear, professional guidance, and a commitment to foot health, you can regain comfort and mobility. Remember, your feet are the unsung heroes of your fitness journey, and investing in their well-being can have a profound impact on your overall health and quality of life.

7. **The Power of Customized Care:** When it comes to foot health, a one-size-fits-all approach may not be ideal. Your feet are as unique as you are, and addressing specific issues requires a personalized approach. That's where a Certified Integrative Movement Specialist can make a significant difference. These experts are trained to assess your body's movement patterns, identify areas of weakness or dysfunction, and develop tailored plans to enhance your overall foot function. Whether you're struggling with balance, mobility, or specific foot issues, a specialist can be your guide on the path to healthier, happier feet.

8. **The Journey to Stronger, Healthier Feet:** The road to foot health may not always be easy, but it's a journey worth

taking. By dedicating time and effort to caring for your feet, you're not only improving your mobility and comfort, but also positively affecting your entire body. Remember, your feet are the foundation of your movement, and when your foundation is solid, everything built upon it is more stable and resilient.

9. **Embrace Foot Freedom:** As discussed earlier, the natural state of your unshod (bare) foot is wide and mobile. Consider spending more time barefoot at home or in environments where it's safe to do so (not on hard surfaces like tile or concrete). This allows your feet to breathe and expand naturally, promoting better circulation and overall foot health.

10. **Stretch and Mobilize:** Incorporate regular light stretching and mobility exercises into your daily routine. Simple exercises like ankle circles, calf stretches, and toe spreads can help maintain flexibility and improve blood flow to your feet.

11. **Mindful Walking:** Pay attention to your walking patterns and posture. Avoid excessive pronation (rolling inward) or supination (rolling outward) of your feet, as these can lead to various foot problems. A Certified Integrative Movement Specialist can provide guidance on improving your gait.

12. **Foot Soaks:** Treat your feet to soothing foot soaks from time to time. Epsom salt foot baths can help relax muscles and ease foot fatigue.

13. **Nutrition and Hydration:** Proper nutrition and hydration are essential for overall health, including that of your feet. Stay

hydrated to maintain circulation, and ensure your diet includes nutrients that support bone and joint health.

14. **Mind-Body Connection:** Remember that your feet are not just physical tools, but also a part of your mind-body connection. Practice mindfulness and relaxation techniques to reduce stress, as excessive stress can manifest physically in your feet.

By incorporating these additional tips and embracing more of a holistic approach to foot health, you can reach a more desirable outcome for maintaining the well-being of your feet. Your feet, after all, are the unsung heroes of your daily life, and caring for them is a worthy investment in your overall health and fitness. Start from the ground up and watch what happens!

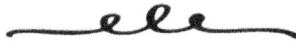

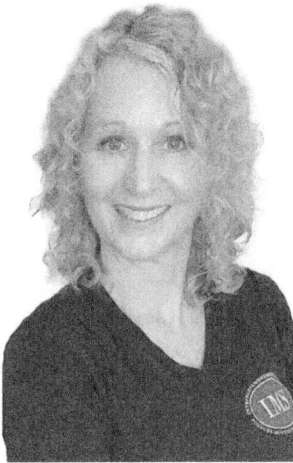

Julie Anne's story really begins as an overweight child. Growing up, she ate sugary foods daily, was sedentary, and was the second largest child in school. As a young adult, Julie Anne was concerned about her weight, so she joined an aerobics class, and it was then, that she fell in love with movement!

Fast forward a few years and 3 children later, Julie Anne still struggled with her weight and sugar addiction. So, she decided to become an aerobics instructor. Shortly thereafter, and for the first time, Julie Anne was finally in control of her weight. Exercise had helped change her life, and she could see how much it benefited her class attendees. Julie Anne wanted to touch individuals on a more intimate level, so she then became a personal trainer.

Now Julie Anne was really helping others strengthen like never before! Every year, she went off to school to learn more so that she could help her clients achieve better results. There was a major problem, though. Julie Anne primarily serves the 50 and above crowd. The information out there was either geared towards the younger generation, or the extreme opposite, involving chair exercises, or it was information that you really couldn't use.

Mostly, classes were about the next best exercise to train a particular body part. Really? How many different ways do you need to work your abs? Meanwhile, Julie Anne's clients were getting older, and although they were getting stronger, they really didn't look any different from what they did when they first had hired her. And they didn't necessarily move better, in fact, they were getting tighter. Julie Anne could not help them through joint issues or various other conditions. It really bothered her because she felt like she had never had enough education. Julie Anne was very frustrated.

Then she met Dr. Evan Osar, the developer of the Integrative Movement System™, which is a very specific process for posture, exercise, and lifestyle changes. Finally, education that made sense, and that actually worked! This is the system that Julie Anne has been trained in and specializes in, to help individuals not only exercise and move more efficiently, but they actually look different. They look better. They feel better. They are stronger and have better balance and stamina. They have better lives. And Julie Anne is finally in a happy place, knowing that she is providing these folks with the best process to longevity!

https://www.callyms.com

Harnessing the Power of Heart Rate Zones: Unleashing Your Potential with Five Heart Rate Zone Workouts

By: Michael Wolfe

Welcome to a world of fitness where understanding your heart rate becomes the key to unlocking your true workout potential. If you've ever felt like your exercise routine could use a boost, the answer lies in the remarkable concept of heart rate zones. Don't worry if this sounds a bit technical at first; we're here to guide you through the ins and outs of heart rate training in the most friendly and informative way possible.

The Heart Rate Zone Breakdown: A Closer Look

Let's get acquainted with the basics before we embark on this heart rate journey. Your heart is your body's engine, and during exercise, it beats faster to pump oxygen and nutrients to your muscles. Your heart rate is a reflection of this activity, and heart rate zones help you understand how intensely your heart is working. Imagine these zones as gears in a car, each designed for a specific purpose. By understanding and targeting these zones, you can tailor your workouts to achieve distinct goals.

Zone 1 – The Cozy Warm-Up Zone

At around 50-60% of your maximum heart rate, this is where you begin your fitness journey. Zone 1 is perfect for warm-ups and cool-downs, gently preparing your body for more intense activity. Think of it as a leisurely stroll – you're getting the blood flowing without breaking a sweat.

Heart Rate Zone 1 Workout Sample

Incorporating Zone 1 into your workout routine is a fantastic way to gently prepare your body for more intense exercise. This zone helps improve blood flow, warms up your muscles, and mentally prepares you for the workout ahead. Here's a sample workout that focuses on Zone 1:

Duration: 10-15 minutes

Equipment: None required

Instructions:

- **Walking Warm-Up:** Begin with a 3-5 minute easy-paced walk. Focus on taking deep breaths and relaxing your body.

- **Dynamic Stretching:** Spend the next 5 minutes incorporating dynamic stretches. Move your body through a range of motions to gently mobilize your joints and muscles. Examples include leg swings, arm circles, hip rotations, and neck tilts.

Zone 2 – The Aerobic Sweet Spot

Ranging from 60-70% of your maximum heart rate, Zone 2 is all about building endurance and burning fat. This zone enhances your cardiovascular fitness, making it ideal for longer, sustained activities. Imagine a comfortable jog – challenging enough to feel the burn, but sustainable in the long run.

Heart Rate Zone 2 Workout Sample

Zone 2 is where you start to build endurance and burn fat efficiently. This zone challenges your cardiovascular fitness while still allowing you to maintain a sustainable effort. Here's a sample workout that focuses on Zone 2:

Duration: 30-40 minutes

Equipment: Any cardio machine (treadmill, stationary bike, elliptical) or outdoor space for running/cycling

Instructions:

- **Warm-Up:** Begin with a 5-10 minute easy-paced jog or brisk walk to get your heart rate slightly elevated.

- **Aerobic Phase:** Increase your intensity to a level where you can still maintain a conversation without gasping for breath. Aim for a heart rate that's around 60-70% of your maximum.

- **Steady-State Effort:** Maintain this intensity for the next 20-30 minutes. You should feel like you're working, but you're not pushing yourself to the limit. Keep your breathing controlled and steady.

- **Variation:** If you're running or cycling, you can vary the terrain or resistance to keep things interesting. For example, include some gentle inclines if you're outdoors, or adjust the resistance on a stationary bike.

- **Cool-Down:** Gradually decrease your intensity and finish with a

5-10 minute easy-paced walk or slow pedaling to bring your heart rate back down.

Suggested Tips:

- Zone 2 workouts are ideal for improving your aerobic capacity and fat-burning efficiency.

- Maintain a consistent pace throughout the workout, aiming to stay within the 60-70% of maximum heart rate range.

- It's normal to break a sweat, but you shouldn't feel out of breath or overly fatigued during Zone 2 workouts.

- If you're using a heart rate monitor, stay mindful of your heart rate to ensure you're staying within the Zone 2 range.

This Zone 2 workout is perfect for individuals looking to build endurance and improve their cardiovascular fitness. It strikes a balance between challenging your body and allowing you to sustain the effort over an extended period. As you progress, you can gradually increase the duration of your Zone 2 workouts or add slight variations to keep things engaging. Remember, consistency is key to reaping the rewards of heart rate zone training.

Zone 3 – The Tempo Zone

As your heart rate reaches 70-80% of your maximum, you're stepping into the tempo zone. This zone pushes your anaerobic threshold, improving your ability to tolerate higher levels of effort. It's like maintaining a brisk pace during a run – you're putting in effort, but you're not gasping for air just yet.

Heart Rate Zone 3 Workout Sample

Zone 3 workouts focus on improving your anaerobic threshold and pushing your body's ability to sustain higher levels of effort. These workouts are challenging but highly effective for increasing your fitness level. Here's a sample workout that targets Zone 3:

Duration: 25-35 minutes

Equipment: Treadmill or outdoor running space

Instructions:

- **Warm-Up:** Start with a 5-10 minute light jog or brisk walk to get your muscles warmed up and your heart rate slightly elevated.

- **Steady Build-Up:** Gradually increase your pace to a level where you can still hold a conversation but your breathing is becoming more controlled and rhythmic.

- **Enter Zone 3:** Once you've found a pace where you're breathing noticeably harder and you're just below the point of breathlessness, you've entered Zone 3. Your heart rate should be around 70-80% of your maximum.

- **Tempo Intervals:** Alternate between 3 minutes in Zone 3 and 1 minute of active recovery (easy jogging or brisk walking). Repeat this cycle for a total of 5 sets.

- **Progressive Finish:** In the last 5 minutes of your workout, gradually increase your pace to the upper end of Zone 3. This will challenge you and simulate a race finish.

- **Cool-Down:** Conclude the workout with a 5-10 minute slow jog or walk to lower your heart rate.

Suggested Tips:

- Zone 3 workouts are intense but manageable. You should feel like you're working hard, but you're able to maintain the effort throughout the workout.

- Focus on your breathing and form. Maintain an efficient stride and keep your chest open for optimal lung capacity.

- It's normal to feel fatigued during Zone 3 workouts, but listen to your body. If you feel excessively out of breath or dizzy, take a break or slow down.

This Zone 3 workout is designed to challenge your cardiovascular system and improve your ability to sustain a moderately high intensity. As you become more comfortable with Zone 3 workouts, you can adjust the interval duration or increase the number of intervals to continue pushing your limits. Consistency in Zone 3 training will lead to improved anaerobic fitness, allowing you to maintain higher intensity efforts for longer durations.

Zone 4 – The Threshold Zone

With your heart rate at 80-90% of your maximum, you're entering the high-intensity territory. Training in Zone 4 enhances your capacity to sustain demanding efforts for more extended periods. Picture yourself doing interval sprints – you're pushing your limits, feeling the burn, and loving the challenge.

Heart Rate Zone 4 Workout Sample

Zone 4 workouts are all about pushing your limits and increasing your ability to sustain high-intensity efforts. These workouts improve your anaerobic capacity and help you tolerate discomfort while maximizing performance gains. Here's a sample Zone 4 workout:

Duration: 20-30 minutes

Equipment: Indoor cycling bike or stationary bike

Instructions:

- **Warm-Up:** Begin with a 5-10 minute easy-paced cycling to warm up your muscles and gradually elevate your heart rate.

- **Build-Up:** Gradually increase the resistance on the bike and start pedaling at a moderate pace. Get your body used to working against resistance.

- **Enter Zone 4:** Once you're ready, increase the resistance even further and start pedaling at an intensity where conversation is difficult. Your heart rate should be around 80-90% of your maximum.

- **Interval Push:** Alternate between 2 minutes in Zone 4 and 1 minute of active recovery (gentle pedaling with lower resistance). Repeat this cycle for a total of 5 sets.

- **Final Push:** In the last 5 minutes, go all out. Push yourself to your maximum effort, mimicking a race finish.

- **Cool-Down:** Conclude the workout with a 5-10 minute easy-paced cycling to gradually lower your heart rate.

Suggested Tips:

- Zone 4 workouts are intense and demanding. You should feel a significant effort and be challenged to maintain the pace.

- Focus on your breathing and maintaining proper cycling form. Keep your core engaged and maintain a smooth pedal stroke.

- If you're using a heart rate monitor, be mindful of your heart rate to ensure you're staying within the Zone 4 range.

This Zone 4 workout is designed to test your limits and enhance your ability to sustain high-intensity efforts. It's ideal for individuals aiming to improve their overall fitness and performance. Remember, Zone 4 workouts should be challenging but sustainable. Listen to your body and adjust the resistance and intensity as needed to ensure a safe and effective workout. Over time, consistent Zone 4 training will lead to improved anaerobic fitness and the ability to maintain higher intensities for longer periods.

Zone 5 – The Maximum Effort Zone

At 90-100% of your max heart rate, you're giving it everything you've got. This zone helps increase your peak performance capacity and truly tests your limits. It's that final sprint in a race where every ounce of energy propels you forward.

Heart Rate Zone 5 Workout Sample

Zone 5 workouts are designed for pushing your body to its limits and maximizing your peak performance capacity. These workouts are highly intense and should be approached with caution. Here's a sample Zone 5 workout:

Duration: 15-20 minutes

Equipment: Treadmill, outdoor space for running, or indoor cycling bike

Instructions:

- **Warm-Up:** Start with a 5-10 minute light jog or brisk walk to warm up your muscles and elevate your heart rate.

- **Build-Up:** Gradually increase your pace to a moderate level where you're starting to feel challenged.

- **Enter Zone 5:** Once you're warmed up, give it your all and push your pace to the absolute maximum effort. Your heart rate should be around 90-100% of your maximum.

- **Maximum Effort Intervals:** Alternate between 30 seconds of maximum effort and 1 minute of complete rest. Repeat this cycle for a total of 5 sets.

- **Cool-Down:** Conclude the workout with a 5-10 minute easy-paced jog or walk to gradually lower your heart rate.

Suggested Tips:

- Zone 5 workouts are extremely demanding and should only be done by individuals with a solid fitness base and familiarity with high-intensity training.

- Listen to your body and stop immediately if you feel lightheaded, dizzy, or excessively fatigued.

- If you're using a heart rate monitor, be cautious about pushing your heart rate to the absolute maximum. Consult with a fitness professional if you're unsure about your maximum heart rate.

Remember that Zone 5 workouts are not meant for everyday training. They are highly intense and should be used sparingly to avoid over-training and potential injury. These workouts are ideal for experienced athletes or individuals with specific performance goals. Always prioritize safety and proper technique when performing Zone 5 workouts.

Harnessing Tools and Technology for Heart Rate Zone Training

In the ever-evolving landscape of fitness, technology has emerged as a valuable ally, offering tools that can enhance your heart rate zone training experience. These tools not only provide real-time feedback but also empower you to personalize your workouts, track progress, and make informed decisions about your training regimen. Let's explore some of the tools and technologies that can take your heart rate zone training to the next level.

- **Heart Rate Monitors and Straps:** Heart rate monitors are one of the cornerstones of heart rate zone training. They provide accurate, real-time data about your heart rate, allowing you to gauge your effort and ensure you're staying within your desired zone. Heart rate straps, worn around the chest, are known for their accuracy and reliability in measuring heart rate. This information helps you tailor your workout intensity to specific zones, maximizing the benefits of each training session.

- **Smartwatches and Fitness Trackers:** Today's smartwatches and fitness trackers have evolved into comprehensive fitness companions. These devices offer heart rate monitoring capabilities, along with additional features like GPS tracking, workout history, and even personalized coaching. Many smartwatches can display your heart rate zones in real-time, making it easier to adjust your effort on the fly and stay in the optimal zone for your goals.

- **Fitness Apps:** There's an app for almost everything, and heart rate zone training is no exception. Fitness apps often integrate with heart rate monitors and smartwatches to provide a wealth of data and analysis. These apps track your workouts, map your heart rate zones, and offer insights into your progress over time. Some apps even generate personalized training plans based on your goals and fitness level.

- **Online Platforms:** Virtual platforms have revolutionized the way we access fitness content. Many online platforms offer heart rate zone-specific workouts led by expert trainers. These sessions guide you through different heart rate zones, ensuring that you're hitting the right intensity levels for optimal results. From indoor cycling classes to interval training, these platforms make heart rate zone training accessible anytime, anywhere.

- **Heart Rate-Responsive Equipment:** The fitness industry has embraced heart rate zone training, leading to the development of heart rate-responsive equipment. These machines adjust resistance or intensity based on your heart rate, guiding you through workouts that automatically adapt to your effort level. This technology ensures you're consistently challenging yourself within your target heart rate zones.

- **Data Analysis and Insights:** Most tools and technologies today offer data analysis features that provide insights into your workouts. From heart rate trends to calorie burn estimates, these insights help you track progress and make informed decisions about your training strategy. Over time, you can see how your fitness is improving as you consistently train within different heart rate zones.

Incorporating tools and technology into your heart rate zone training adds a layer of precision and customization to your fitness journey. Whether you're aiming to lose weight, improve endurance, or enhance overall performance, these tools offer the guidance and feedback needed to optimize your workouts. As you embrace the advantages of technology, remember that these tools are most effective when used in tandem with your own awareness of your body's signals and cues.

Customizing Your Zone-Based Workout Strategy

Now that you're acquainted with the heart rate zones, it's time to put them into practice. A well-rounded workout plan involves a combination of these zones to cater to your specific fitness goals. Whether you're aiming for fat loss, improved endurance, or enhanced speed, each zone plays a vital role in your routine.

Begin your workout with a dynamic warm-up that eases you into Zone 1. Gradually progress through the zones, focusing on the specific goals of your session. This could mean mixing Zone 2, 3, and 4 workouts, depending on what you're aiming to achieve. Always remember, while pushing your boundaries is commendable, overexertion can lead to setbacks. Listen to your body, find your sweet spot, and stay safe.

The Heart Rate Zone Advantage: Transforming Your Fitness Journey

By now, you're armed with the knowledge to revolutionize your workouts. Heart rate zones are like the secret code to unlocking your full fitness potential. They provide structure, guidance, and the promise of a more efficient, effective workout routine. Embracing heart rate training means you're no longer just going through the motions – you're working smarter and more strategically.

So, go ahead and embrace the power of heart rate zones. Whether you're a seasoned athlete or just starting your fitness journey, this concept will elevate your workouts to new heights. As you continue to fine-tune your training and learn to embrace each zone's unique benefits, you'll find that your heart is not only pumping blood but also driving you closer to your fitness aspirations.

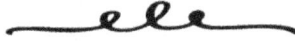

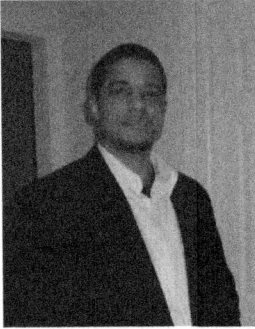

Michael is a professional health and fitness coach with over 20 years in the health industry. He began as a medic in the US ARMY at the age of 18. During his ten years of military service, Michael worked as a combat medic, physical therapy specialist, and medical instructor. His work included the clinical, hospital, and field environments. He aided in the treatment of over 3,000 military servicemen, military family members, DOD workers, US dignitaries, and associates of the US military. This work included overseas medical assignments in South Korean and Iraqi medical centers.

After honorably serving in the US ARMY, Michael began work in the intensive care unit and emergency room. His focus in the intensive care unit was as a physical therapy tech. At 5 a.m., several times a week, he would assist nurses with the movement protocol of patients ranging from stroke victims to post-operative patients recovering from major heart surgery. The work was very intensive and required careful attention to detail. Eventually, Michael made his way to the emergency room as an emergency room tech. He was always on the go assisting doctors and nurses with various patient needs. EKGs, IV setup, and blood draws were the core responsibilities on an hourly basis. Wound care, splinting, catheter setups, and basic triage were also a part of his responsibilities.

Michael began his career as a personal trainer in 2007. He briefly worked in two corporate gym chains. Eventually, he created two fitness training companies. He trains clients online and offline between the Midwest and West Coast with a small support staff. He has helped clients aged 8 to 75 improve their physical well-being and personal performance. His core clientele has been youth athletes, busy professionals, and middle-aged achievers.

The primary training system he swears by is the LEANER STRONGER FASTER SYSTEM™. LEANER means lean eating and nutrition equals results. STRONGER means strength to realize our natural greatness equals results. FASTER means functional and specific training equals results. With this system, he can literally guarantee results as long as each client is compliant and diligent. His thorough approach to each client is influenced by his unique military medical experience and continuous focus on education. He holds certifications as a Master Fitness Trainer through the International Sports Science Association, an Elite Fitness Trainer through the National Academy of Sports Medicine, a Certified Health Coach through the Institute for Integrative Nutrition, and several other respected associations. Michael studied Exercise Science at McNeese State for a year and a half. Prior to this, he completed all his military medical training in Fort Sam Houston, Texas. Here, he completed two medical training programs: a combat medic specialist program - taught by military medical staff and a physical therapy specialist program - designed and led by a Ph.D. in Physical Therapy.

Connect with Michael at PushAndPullPerformance.com or Michael@PushAndPullPerformance.com

Beyond the Binge: Breaking Free From The Cycle of Emotional Eating

By: Mary Ann Bianchini

Imagine a world where every bite you take is driven by true hunger, not by the highs and lows of your emotions. A world where you have the power to enjoy food as nourishment, not as a crutch for your feelings. This is the journey we're about to embark on – a journey beyond the binge, where we break free from the cycle of emotional eating and rediscover a wholesome relationship with food and ourselves.

Understanding Emotional Eating: Peeling Back the Layers

Let's start by peeling back the layers of emotional eating. It's like a dance between your heart and your plate, where emotions often take the lead. Those times when stress, sadness, or even celebration lead us straight to the pantry – that's emotional eating. It's not just about physical hunger; it's about seeking comfort and escape in food.

We've all been there, right? A tough day at work, a fight with a loved one, or even boredom can trigger the urge to reach for a bag of chips or a tub of ice cream. It's like food becomes a friend that listens without judgment. But here's the catch: relying on food to soothe emotions can become a slippery slope, leading to guilt, shame, and a cycle that's tough to break.

The Why Behind the Chew: Unlocking Emotional Eating's Mysteries

Ever wondered why that slice of pizza seems to hold all the answers when you're down? It's not just about the taste; it's about the science behind the scenes. Emotional eating taps into the brain's reward system, releasing feel-good chemicals that temporarily alleviate negative emotions. This creates a strong connection between certain foods and emotional relief.

The mind-body connection also plays a role. Our emotions can influence our sense of taste and even our perception of fullness. That's why when you're feeling blue, those indulgent treats feel extra appealing. Unraveling the mystery of emotional eating helps us gain awareness of how our emotions and biology intertwine to create those intense cravings.

Finding Healthy Coping Strategies: Navigating Negative Emotions

Negative emotions are a part of life, but how we handle them can make all the difference. Enter the world of healthy coping strategies – alternatives to using food as an emotional escape. From journaling and meditation to going for a walk, these strategies empower us to navigate negative emotions without falling into the food trap.

You know those times when stress hits hard, and your immediate reaction is to grab a bag of chips? By recognizing these triggers, you're taking the first step toward breaking free. Journaling your thoughts and feelings can help you unpack the emotions behind those cravings. It's like putting your emotions on paper, allowing you to gain clarity and understanding.

Feeding the Soul: Exploring the Roots of Emotional Hunger

We all have our reasons for emotional eating – it's like diving into the past to understand the present. Exploring the roots of emotional hunger is like embarking on a journey to understand why certain emotions trigger specific food cravings. These cravings can stem from memories, cultural influences, and even childhood experiences.

For instance, that bowl of chicken soup might remind you of comforting moments with your family when you were young. Understanding these connections gives you the power to make conscious choices. You can still enjoy those comfort foods, but now you're aware of why they hold such a special place in your heart and taste buds.

Embracing Self-Compassion: Overcoming Guilt and Shame

Guilt and shame often accompany emotional eating, creating a vicious cycle that's tough to escape. But here's the thing – there's no need to beat yourself up. It's time to embrace self-compassion and understand that emotional eating is a normal response to life's challenges. By acknowledging your emotions without judgment, you're taking a giant step toward breaking free from guilt and shame.

Imagine this: instead of berating yourself for indulging in that dessert, you pause and remind yourself that it's okay to have these moments. Self-compassion is about treating yourself with kindness and understanding, just as you would a friend. This gentle approach not only helps you break free from the guilt-shame cycle but also nurtures a positive relationship with yourself.

Mindful Eating: Listening to Your Body's True Hunger Cues

Mindful eating is like a superpower that helps you regain control over your relationship with food. It's about tuning into your body's signals, understanding when you're truly hungry, and recognizing when emotions are at play. Mindful eating encourages you to savor each bite, cultivating a deeper appreciation for the nourishment that food provides.

Picture this: you're sitting down to a meal, savoring the flavors, textures, and aromas. You're not just eating; you're experiencing the meal with all your senses. Mindful eating also encourages you to listen to your body's cues of fullness. This means you're less likely to overeat because you're attuned to when your body has had enough. It's like forming a harmonious partnership between your emotions and your plate.

Breaking Free: Strategies to Disrupt the Cycle of Emotional Eating

Breaking free from the cycle of emotional eating requires a toolkit of strategies to disrupt the patterns that have held you captive. By recognizing your triggers, you're able to interrupt the automatic response of reaching for food when emotions surge. This is your chance to implement those healthy coping techniques you've been learning – from taking a walk to practicing deep breathing.

Imagine this: you're in the middle of a stressful day, and instead of reaching for a candy bar, you decide to step outside for a brisk walk. As you walk, you focus on your breath and let the fresh air clear your mind. By choosing this strategy, you're breaking the chain of emotional eating and finding a healthier way to manage stress.

Savoring Life: Embracing Nourishment Beyond Food

Life is a tapestry woven with experiences, relationships, and moments of joy. Embracing nourishment beyond food means recognizing that fulfillment comes from a variety of sources. It's about finding joy in hobbies, spending time with loved ones, and engaging in activities that light up your soul. When you create a well-rounded life, emotional eating loses its grip.

Imagine this: instead of turning to food for comfort, you reach out to a friend for a heart-to-heart conversation. You both share laughter and support, leaving you with a sense of emotional nourishment that transcends what any snack could provide. Embracing nourishment beyond food is like opening the door to a world of fulfillment that extends far beyond the plate.

Breaking Free: Your Journey to Wholeness

As you journey through the realms of emotional eating, you're not just breaking free from a cycle; you're embarking on a journey to wholeness. By understanding the complexities of emotional eating, you're reclaiming the power to make mindful choices that honor your emotions and well-being. It's about fostering a kinder relationship with yourself, recognizing that your feelings are valid, and finding healthier ways to navigate them.

Imagine a life where food is a source of nourishment, pleasure, and celebration – where emotions are acknowledged and managed without relying on food as a crutch. This is the vision of a life beyond the binge, a life where you've broken free from the chains of emotional eating and embraced a path of empowerment and growth. So, are you ready to take the leap?

Breaking Free: Your Journey to Wholeness

As you journey through the realms of emotional eating, you're not just breaking free from a cycle; you're embarking on a journey to wholeness. By understanding the complexities of emotional eating, you're reclaiming the power to make mindful choices that honor your emotions and well-being. It's about fostering a kinder relationship with yourself, recognizing that your feelings are valid, and finding healthier ways to navigate them.

Imagine a life where food is a source of nourishment, pleasure, and celebration – where emotions are acknowledged and managed without relying on food as a crutch. This is the vision of a life beyond the binge, a life where you've broken free from the chains of emotional eating and embraced a path of empowerment and growth. So, are you ready to take the leap? The journey to breaking free from the cycle of emotional eating is a transformative one, filled with self-discovery, compassion, and a newfound sense of control.

Remember, you're not alone on this journey. You have the tools, insights, and strategies to navigate the ups and downs. You've uncovered the secrets of emotional eating, dug deep into your triggers, and learned to cope in healthier ways. You've embraced self-compassion and mindfulness, strengthening the connection between your emotions and your plate.

With each step you take, you're rewriting your relationship with food and emotions. You're creating a life where food serves its purpose – nourishing your body – and emotions find their place in a tapestry of experiences. The road ahead might have its challenges, but armed with knowledge and determination, you're equipped to overcome them.

So, here's to breaking free – to a life of balance, self-love, and empowerment. It's not just about letting go of emotional eating; it's about embracing a journey that leads you to a place of wholeness and well-being. As you move forward, remember that every choice you make is a step toward a brighter, healthier future. You're the author of your own story, and this chapter is just the beginning of the incredible journey that lies ahead. Let's keep moving forward, breaking free from the cycle of emotional eating, and embracing a life beyond the binge.

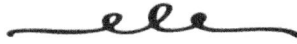

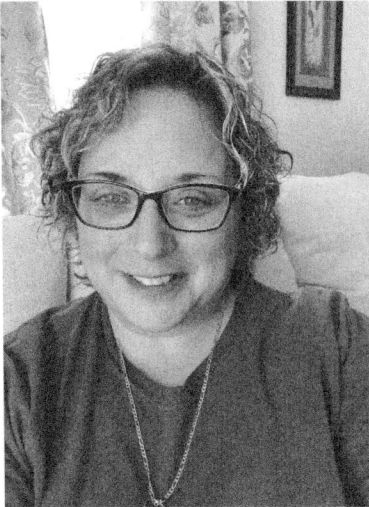

Born and raised in Cleveland, Ohio, Mary Ann Bianchini is the youngest of four children. Being raised in an Italian family, food was a major part of everything about her heritage. Breakfast, dinner, family gatherings, holidays, funerals, even for no reason in particular... EVERYTHING involved copious amounts of food.

When life threw a major curve ball, food was Mary Ann's solace, her comforter. Food was her escape from reality.

Until she acknowledged her unhealthy relationship with food, she was on a never-ending and self-depreciating cycle of guilt-ridden overindulgence with food. Unhappy with the events in her life and how they always led to food, Mary Ann decided to make a radical change to her life.

To this day, Mary Ann will tell you... amazing things happen on the other side of change!

Mary Ann has spent years studying the mind-body connection as well as receiving a certification in the psychology of emotional eating. Her program, which uses simple solutions to eliminate the vicious cycle of emotional eating, has helped hundreds of women create a healthier relationship with food along with finding the joy in life that has been missing.

Mary Ann's newest book, **"Beyond the Binge: Breaking Free From The Cycle of Emotional Eating,"** goes into much more details and provides the exact blueprint for breaking free from the never-ending cycle of emotional eating and taking control of the life you deserve. You can grab his book for yourself at **https://mailchi.mp/5048ecf062a9/bdnrelv4nk**.

gethookedfitness@yahoo.com

Navigating Diabetes: Seniors' Comprehensive Blueprint for Success

By: Najiy Q. Asaad

Embarking on the journey of managing diabetes in your senior years may seem like a challenging task, but armed with the right knowledge, practical strategies, and a positive mindset, you can navigate this path with confidence and resilience. In this comprehensive guide, "Navigating Diabetes: Seniors' Comprehensive Blueprint for Success," we delve into the intricate world of diabetes management for seniors, offering you a comprehensive toolkit to empower you on your journey to health, vitality, and fulfillment.

Understanding Diabetes in Seniors: The Foundation of Success

As you set out on this journey, understanding the fundamental aspects of diabetes is paramount. For seniors, managing diabetes comes with unique considerations. Regular health check-ups, diligent blood sugar monitoring, and recognizing the subtle warning signs become essential habits to maintain optimal health. The changes that come with aging can impact your diabetes, making it crucial to stay vigilant and proactive about your well-being.

Building a Strong Support System: Your Pillar of Strength

Managing diabetes isn't a solo mission – it's a collaborative effort. Building a strong support system is pivotal for emotional well-being and successful diabetes management. Communicating openly with family, friends, and healthcare professionals ensures you're never alone on this journey. Don't underestimate the power of diabetes support groups – these connections provide a space to share experiences, gain insights, and foster a sense of belonging.

Eating Well for Diabetes Management: Fueling Your Wellness

Your diet plays a central role in your diabetes journey. Embracing a balanced, nutrient-rich diet is crucial for blood sugar control. Incorporate whole grains, lean proteins, colorful vegetables, fruits, and healthy fats into your meals. Opt for frequent, smaller meals to prevent blood sugar spikes and crashes. By crafting a meal plan that aligns with your tastes and dietary needs, you'll enjoy a satisfying and diabetes-friendly diet.

Here's a sample 3-day meal plan designed to help control diabetes. Remember that individual dietary needs may vary, so it's essential to work with a healthcare professional or registered dietitian to create a meal plan that suits your specific requirements.

Day 1:

Breakfast:

- Scrambled eggs with spinach and tomatoes

- Whole-grain toast

- A small bowl of mixed berries

Lunch:

- Grilled chicken salad with mixed greens, cucumbers, bell peppers, and a light vinaigrette dressing

- A small apple

Snack:

- Carrot and celery sticks with hummus

Dinner:

- Baked salmon with a lemon-dill sauce

- Steamed broccoli

- Quinoa

Day 2:

Breakfast:

- Greek yogurt with chopped walnuts and a sprinkle of cinnamon

- Sliced strawberries

Lunch:

- Turkey and avocado wrap in a whole-grain tortilla

- Mixed baby carrots

Snack:

- Handful of almonds

Dinner:

- Grilled lean steak

- Roasted Brussels sprouts

- Cauliflower mashed "potatoes"

Day 3:

Breakfast:

- Oatmeal topped with sliced bananas and a drizzle of almond butter

- Herbal tea or black coffee (if desired)

Lunch:

- Lentil soup

- Side salad with mixed greens, cherry tomatoes, and a light vinaigrette

Snack:

- Cottage cheese with pineapple chunks

Dinner:

- Stir-fried tofu with broccoli, bell peppers, and snap peas in a light soy-ginger sauce

- Brown rice

General Tips for Diabetes-Friendly Meals:

Choose Whole Grains: Opt for whole-grain options like brown rice, quinoa, whole-grain bread, and whole-wheat pasta to help regulate blood sugar levels.

Prioritize Lean Proteins: Incorporate lean proteins such as chicken, turkey, fish, tofu, legumes, and low-fat dairy to support muscle health and stabilize blood sugar.

Embrace Fiber: Include plenty of fiber-rich foods like vegetables, fruits, whole grains, and legumes. Fiber aids digestion and helps manage blood sugar spikes.

Healthy Fats: Include sources of healthy fats such as avocados, nuts, seeds, and olive oil in moderation.

Portion Control: Pay attention to portion sizes to avoid overeating and help manage blood sugar levels.

Limit Added Sugars: Minimize or avoid sugary foods and beverages. Opt for natural sweeteners like fruit to satisfy your sweet cravings.

Stay Hydrated: Drink plenty of water throughout the day to stay hydrated and support overall health.

Remember that everyone's nutritional needs are unique. It's essential to work closely with your healthcare provider or a registered dietitian to tailor a meal plan that aligns with your specific health goals, lifestyle, and preferences. Regular monitoring of blood sugar levels and adjustments to your meal plan can help you achieve and maintain optimal diabetes management.

Staying Active and Fit: Energizing Your Body

Physical activity is a cornerstone of diabetes management for seniors. Engaging in regular exercise not only regulates blood sugar levels but also enhances cardiovascular health, flexibility, and overall well-being. Delve into age-appropriate exercises, prioritize daily movement, and consider low-impact options like walking, swimming, or gentle yoga. Embracing an active lifestyle infuses energy into your days and contributes to your overall health.

Here's a sample 3-week workout program designed for seniors that emphasizes age-appropriate exercises, daily movement, and low-impact options like walking. As always, consult with your healthcare provider before beginning any new exercise program, especially if you have underlying health conditions.

Week 1: Getting Started

Note: Perform each exercise for 10-15 repetitions (reps) and 1-2 sets. Start with a warm-up of 5-10 minutes of light walking or marching in place.

Day 1:

- **Walking:** 20-30 minutes of brisk walking in your neighborhood or a local park.

- **Standing Leg Raises:** Hold onto a sturdy surface if needed. Lift one leg to the side, front, and back for 10-15 reps on each leg.

- **Seated March:** Sit on a sturdy chair and march your legs in place for 1-2 minutes.

Day 2:

- **Gentle Yoga or Stretching:** Focus on gentle stretches for flexibility and relaxation.

- **Arm Circles:** Stand or sit with arms extended to the sides. Make small circles forward and then backward for 10-15 reps.

Day 3:

- **Walking:** 20-30 minutes of brisk walking.

- **Wall Push-Ups:** Stand arm's length away from a wall. Place your hands on the wall at chest height and do push-ups against the wall for 10-15 reps.

Week 2: Increasing Intensity

Note: Continue with the warm-up routine and increase exercise intensity by adding more reps or sets.

Day 1:

- **Walking:** 20-30 minutes of brisk walking.

- **Chair Squats:** Sit on a chair and stand up without using your hands. Lower back down slowly for 10-15 reps.

Day 2:

- **Gentle Yoga or Stretching:** Focus on deeper stretches to improve flexibility.

- **Toe Taps:** Sit on a chair and tap your toes on the floor alternately for 1-2 minutes.

Day 3:

- **Walking:** 20-30 minutes of brisk walking.

- **Leg Extensions:** Sit on a chair and extend one leg straight out in front of you. Lower it back down and switch legs for 10-15 reps on each leg.

Week 3: Adding Variety

Note: Continue with the warm-up routine and consider adding light hand weights (1-2 pounds) for resistance.

Day 1:

- **Walking:** 20-30 minutes of brisk walking.

- **Standing Heel Raises:** Stand behind a chair for support. Raise your heels off the ground and lower them back down for 10-15 reps.

Day 2:

- **Gentle Yoga or Stretching:** Focus on a mix of stretches to improve flexibility and balance.

- **Seated Row:** Sit on a chair and hold light weights. Pull the weights towards your chest, squeezing your shoulder blades together, for 10-15 reps.

Day 3:

- **Walking:** 20-30 minutes of brisk walking.

- **Side Leg Lifts:** Hold onto a chair for support. Lift one leg to the side and lower it back down for 10-15 reps on each leg.

Remember to listen to your body and modify exercises as needed. Consistency is key to seeing progress, so aim to incorporate daily movement into your routine. Staying active helps improve cardiovascular health, maintain muscle strength, and enhance overall well-being.

Managing Medications and Insulin: Navigating Treatment

Effective management of medications and insulin is pivotal for diabetes control. Creating a structured medication schedule ensures consistency and precision in your treatment plan. Effective communication with your healthcare providers is essential for addressing concerns, making adjustments, and ensuring your medications align with your evolving health needs. Regularly review your medication plan to accommodate changes in your health or lifestyle.

Stress Reduction and Emotional Well-being: Nurturing Your Mind

Stress can wield a significant impact on blood sugar levels. Integrating relaxation techniques, meditation practices, and stress management strategies into your daily routine is a proactive approach to emotional well-being. Prioritize your mental health, engage in activities that spark joy, and surround yourself with positive influences. Cultivating emotional resilience is a cornerstone of thriving with diabetes.

Foot Care and Skin Health: Navigating Potential Complications

Seniors managing diabetes should pay special attention to foot care and skin health. Regular foot inspections, proper footwear choices, and meticulous skincare routines are key preventive measures. Routine visits to a podiatrist for professional foot care can help you avoid complications. By tending to your skin and feet, you're taking proactive steps towards overall health.

Coping with Common Diabetes Complications: A Comprehensive Approach

Proactively addressing potential complications is crucial for seniors managing diabetes. Regular eye and dental exams, effective neuropathy management, and prioritizing heart health through diet, exercise, and medication are vital aspects of your journey. By staying informed and proactive, you're empowered to manage complications and preserve your overall well-being.

Traveling and Socializing with Diabetes: Embracing Life's Adventures

Seniors deserve to relish life's adventures and social connections, even while managing diabetes. Preparing for travel, packing diabetes essentials, and making informed choices while dining out are strategies that empower you to embrace life's experiences. Open communication about dietary needs, making mindful choices, and weaving physical activity into your travel plans and social gatherings enable you to create cherished memories.

Creating a Sustainable Diabetes Lifestyle: Forging Your Path to Success

Creating a sustainable diabetes lifestyle amalgamates all the insights and strategies we've explored thus far. By setting SMART goals, crafting a structured daily routine, maintaining a balanced diet, engaging in physical activity, and nurturing a robust support system, you're sculpting a life of wellness. Embrace flexibility, celebrate each step of progress, and prioritize self-care as you navigate your diabetes journey with unwavering resilience and a sense of purpose.

In closing, "Navigating Diabetes: Seniors' Comprehensive Blueprint for Success" is your steadfast companion on your journey towards thriving with diabetes in your golden years. Armed with knowledge and practical strategies, you're well-equipped to manage diabetes effectively, relish a life of fulfillment, and seize each day as an opportunity to flourish. Your diabetes journey is a testament to your strength and tenacity – here's to a future brimming with health, happiness, and endless possibilities.

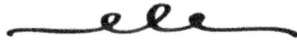

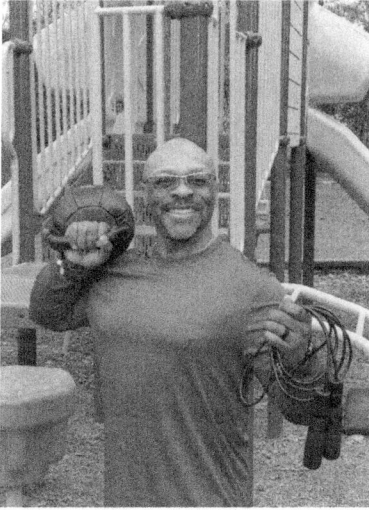

A fitness professional with 22+ years of experience, Naajiy Q. Asaad (aka Coach "G") is a proud military veteran that works with seniors and beginners who want to jumpstart their fitness goals, build strength, boost stamina, manage their weight, and increase their mobility and flexibility!

As a Senior Fitness Specialist and Type II Diabetic Fitness Specialist, Naajiy's main goal is to help his clients achieve their personal fitness goals and lead a healthy lifestyle. He is committed to building lifelong professional relationships with his clients and using the most effective fitness techniques and programs to produce results as quickly as possible.

Naajiy is dedicated to staying up-to-date with the latest fitness advancements through continuing education so that he can incorporate the most modern and effective fitness tools to improve his clients' strength, endurance, flexibility, and overall physique. He follows scientifically proven protocols to help his clients achieve their fitness goals as efficiently as possible.

Naajiy creates simple, and highly effective plans that can help you reach your goals from anywhere. Whether you need help in the gym, at home, or with healthy recipe ideas, he's got you covered.

As a Type II Diabetic Fitness Specialist and Senior Fitness Coach with 20+ years of experience, Naajiy can help you to feel and look like the greatest version of YOURSELF again. Yes, he's here to help you get your SWAG back!

Naajiy's newest book, "**Navigating Diabetes: Seniors' Comprehensive Blueprint for Success**," goes into much more details and provides the exact blueprint for savoring the joys of family, pursuing passions, and cherishing the fruits of decades well-lived despite the challenges of managing diabetes. You can grab his book for yourself at https://www.fitandtrimuniversity.com/navigating-diabetes.

www.FitandTrimUniversity.com

Hormone Secrets: Decoding the Hidden Messages of Your Body

By: Dr. Bobby Muniz

Embracing the Melodies of Change: A Woman's Journey Through Hormones and Menopause

Once upon a time, in a quaint town nestled between rolling hills and tranquil lakes, lived a woman named Eleanor. Eleanor was in her early 50s, a point in life where she had already weathered the storms of youth and the challenges of adulthood. However, a new chapter was unfolding—one that she hadn't fully anticipated—the chapter of menopause.

Eleanor had always been an active and vibrant soul, but as the years went by, she began to notice changes within her body and mind. Sleepless nights replaced restful slumber, her moods danced like leaves in the wind, and she felt an unexplained warmth spreading through her body. Confused and curious, Eleanor decided it was time to decipher the hidden messages her body was sending her.

One morning, as the golden sun painted the sky, Eleanor embarked on a journey of discovery. Armed with books, conversations with friends, and a newfound sense of determination, she set out to navigate the intricate realm of hormones and menopause. She realized that her body was going through a transformative phase, where the orchestra of hormones that had accompanied her for decades was now playing a different tune.

As Eleanor delved into the world of menopause, she learned about the waltz of estrogen and progesterone, once steadfast partners in her monthly cycle. With aging, their dance was fading, leading to the symphony of changes she was experiencing. Armed with knowledge, Eleanor embraced self-care as a new mantra. She began practicing mindfulness, exploring yoga, and rediscovering the joy of creative expression.

But Eleanor's journey wasn't just about the physical changes—she was also uncovering the emotional aspects of menopause. She realized that her moods were like waves, sometimes crashing and sometimes gentle. With the support of friends who had already walked this path, she learned to ride these emotional tides with grace, reaching out for understanding and connection during the tougher moments.

One pivotal moment on Eleanor's journey came during a retreat by the serene lakeside. As the moon cast a shimmering path on the water, Eleanor gathered around a bonfire with other women, all at various stages of life's journey. Here, under the twinkling stars, they shared stories—of laughter, of tears, and of the wisdom they had gleaned from their own hormonal symphonies.

Listening to these stories, Eleanor realized that her journey was not isolated; it was a rite of passage that countless women had navigated before her. She felt the strength of this sisterhood, of women who had embraced the hidden messages of their hormones, emerged wiser, and continued to live life vibrantly.

With newfound clarity and a heart full of resilience, Eleanor continued her journey. She embraced each change, each message her body was sending her, as a note in her own unique symphony. She found solace in the present moment, and in doing so, discovered a serenity she hadn't known before.

Years later, as Eleanor looked back on her journey, she marveled at the beauty of it all—the highs and lows, the laughter and tears. She had not only decoded the hidden messages of her hormones and menopause, but had also uncovered a newfound appreciation for her body and its ever-growing nature.

And so, Eleanor's story became a melody of courage, wisdom, and growth. Her journey through hormones and menopause had transformed her into a woman who danced to her own rhythm, embracing every note that life's symphony had to offer.

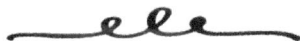

Every day, within the intricate confines of your body, an incredible symphony is performed—a symphony composed and conducted by hormones. These silent messengers are the invisible architects of your health, orchestrating a harmonious dance of emotions, metabolism, growth, and much more. Welcome to the enlightening odyssey of "Hormone Secrets: Decoding the Hidden Messages of Your Body," where we embark on a journey to unlock the profound influence of hormones on your well-being, unravel their mysteries, and discover how they guide your life's melody.

The Dance of Hormonal Balance and Imbalance

Imagine your body as a finely tuned orchestra, with hormones acting as the maestros conducting a delicate dance of equilibrium. The symphony begins in the endocrine system—an intricate network of glands scattered throughout your body. Picture these glands as musicians, each playing their unique melody to contribute to the harmony of your health.

However, life's rhythm isn't always steady. Stress, lifestyle factors, and external influences can create dissonance in this symphony. Hormonal imbalance emerges as mood swings, energy slumps, and weight fluctuations. This is where the importance of hormonal harmony becomes clear. Embracing strategies like self-care, balanced nutrition, and stress management helps bring back the harmonious melody to your life's composition.

Crafting a Balanced Lifestyle for Hormonal Equilibrium

Picture your lifestyle as the conductor of your hormonal symphony. Your choices—ranging from what you eat to how you sleep—resonate within your body, either harmonizing with its needs or creating discord.

Balanced nutrition isn't merely a trend—it's the sustenance your hormones require to functioning optimally. Think of lean proteins, vibrant vegetables, and nourishing fats as the harmonious ensemble of health. Exercise takes center stage too, invigorating your mood, enhancing insulin sensitivity, and fostering hormonal balance.

And then there's sleep, the star player in your well-being. Quality rest provides your body with the opportunity to recalibrate, boosting growth hormone production, regulating appetite hormones, and even enhancing your emotional equilibrium.

Unveiling the Mysteries of Puberty

Remember the tumultuous journey of adolescence—the hormonal roller coaster that led to physical and emotional transformations? Welcome to the enigma of puberty, a chapter where sex hormones such as estrogen and testosterone sculpt your body and emotions, transforming you from child to adult.

As girls experience the blossoming of breasts and the onset of menstruation, estrogen orchestrates these changes. Boys, on the other hand, witness voice deepening, facial hair growth, and muscle development, all guided by the baton of testosterone. By understanding these hormonal shifts, we can support young individuals navigating these changes, fostering open conversations and providing knowledge for an empowered journey.

Navigating the Waters of Menopause

As the chapters of life unfold, women enter the realm of menopause—a transformative phase. Estrogen levels ebb, leading to hot flashes, mood fluctuations, and shifts in bone health. Though it's not without challenges, understanding this chapter empowers women to navigate it with grace and confidence.

Through knowledge, supportive communities, and self-care practices, this phase of life can be embraced as a liberating experience rather than a daunting one. By decoding the hormonal nuances of menopause, women can journey through it with resilience and celebrate the wisdom it brings.

The Stress Hormone: Unveiling the Mind-Body Connection

Stress—a modern-day specter—plays a role far more profound than we often acknowledge. Enter cortisol, the stress hormone, orchestrating the fight-or-flight response. In measured doses, cortisol is a protector. However, chronic stress transforms it into a discordant tune within your symphony.

The mind-body connection becomes clear as stress disrupts hormonal balance. Cortisol surges increase appetite, potentially leading to weight gain. Sleep disturbances arise, affecting growth hormone production. This chapter underscores the importance of stress management—practices like mindfulness, meditation, and physical activity become essential notes in rewriting this hormonal melody.

Fertility: The Intricate Hormonal Dance of Reproduction

Life's symphony continues with fertility—an intricate dance of hormones that prepare your body for the creation of life. It's not solely about timing; it's about hormonal harmony, orchestrating conception, and nurturing a pregnancy.

Here, we unravel the hormonal ballet of the menstrual cycle—the rise and fall of estrogen and progesterone preparing the uterine lining for potential pregnancy. The role of male hormones like testosterone in male fertility also comes into play. Understanding these hormonal cues empowers individuals and couples to make informed choices about family planning.

The Melody of Weight and Metabolism

Weight management isn't just about calories in and calories out; it's a hormonal melody where metabolism takes center stage. Insulin, the gatekeeper of glucose, influences fat storage. Leptin, your satiety hormone, signals fullness. Ghrelin, the hunger hormone, alerts you to hunger.

Fad diets stumble when faced with the complexity of hormones. Instead, nurturing your body with balanced nutrition, mindful eating, and regular physical activity creates a harmonious hormonal environment, fostering sustainable weight management.

Harmony of Happiness: Serotonin, Oxytocin, and Emotional Well-Being

Hormones aren't confined to the realm of the physical; they're architects of your emotions too. Serotonin, the happiness hormone, paints joy across your emotional canvas. Oxytocin, the love hormone, fosters bonds and trust.

By engaging in self-care, nurturing relationships, and adopting a positive mindset, you can optimize the release of these friendly hormones, creating a life of emotional well-being and connection.

Aging Gracefully: Hormonal Insights for Vitality

The passage of time brings with it the symphony of aging, where experience blends with newfound wisdom. This chapter, like the overture to a magnificent composition, introduces us to the harmonies of hormonal vitality that guide us through the later stages of life.

Imagine this phase as a richly textured piece, with hormones serving as the orchestra's conductors. While the notes might change, the harmonious ensemble remains, influencing energy levels, emotional well-being, and connections to others. Estrogen, despite its shift, continues to safeguard bone and heart health, while testosterone quietly sustains energy and muscle tone.

Hormones extend beyond the physical; they shape the emotional landscape as well. Serotonin paints the canvas of your life with joy, while oxytocin fosters connections that enrich your journey. Grasping these emotional nuances, you can nurture relationships, practice self-care, and embrace gratitude to create a harmonious emotional symphony.

As the conductor of this symphony of aging, self-care takes center stage. Exercise not only maintains physical strength but also triggers the release of endorphins, nature's mood enhancers. Nutrient-rich foods fuel your body's hormonal harmonies, sustaining both vitality and well-being. Prioritizing quality sleep, your body's natural intermission, ensures the rejuvenation brought about by growth hormone.

Wisdom arises from navigating changes with grace. The shift brought by menopause, while altering estrogen's role, leaves behind immeasurable wisdom. It's a time to celebrate your journey's resilience, shared laughter, and connections forged. Your hormonal symphony becomes a unique and beautiful melody, embracing its ebb and flow to weave the tapestry of your life.

As you journey through the years, remember that you hold the baton. Guided by insights from your body's hormonal symphony, you craft a life of depth, well-being, and vitality. Aging becomes a composition of grace, wisdom, and the enduring harmonies that continue to shape your path. Just as an orchestra matures and deepens its sound, so does your understanding of hormones and their roles, creating a symphony of life well-lived.

Beyond Biology: Social and Environmental Influences

The final movement explores the broader context of hormonal health. Social connections, self-care practices, and the environment interact with your hormones, affecting your overall well-being.

Nurturing positive relationships, practicing self-care, and embracing a healthy environment create a harmonious melody that resonates with balance, vitality, and inner peace.

Conclusion: A Lifelong Journey with Hormone Secrets

And so, dear reader, you've embarked on an intricate journey through the realm of hormones. From balance to imbalances, from the rhythms of puberty to the symphony of menopause, hormones are the concealed conductors of your life's music.

Remember, you wield the baton to this symphony. Empowered with knowledge, understanding, and friendly strategies, you orchestrate a life of vitality, well-being, and harmony. Embrace your body's wisdom, nurture your hormonal symphony, and allow it to guide you toward a life of health and happiness. The secrets of hormones are now unveiled, and it's up to you to decode them, tune your life, and let the harmonious melodies resonate through every aspect of your being.

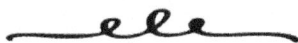

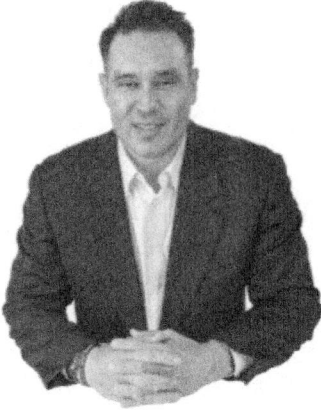

With an impressive career spanning over a decade in the sphere of functional medicine, Dr. Bobby Muñiz stands out as an accomplished and trusted professional. His vast expertise and unrivaled commitment have enabled him to guide countless individuals towards optimal hormonal balance and overall health improvement. The prestige of his fellowship from the American Academy of Anti-Aging further attests to his proficiency in his chosen field, solidifying his reputation as a well-qualified expert.

In addition to his work in medicine, Dr. Muñiz has been an influential figure within the Harlingen CISD Board of Trustees since his inauguration in June 2014. His leadership skills were recognized by the Texas Association of School Boards, which selected him for the Leadership TASB Class of 2017.

A native of Harlingen, Texas, Dr. Muñiz proudly graduated from Harlingen High School in 1992. His educational roots can be traced back to Treasure Hills Elementary and Coakley Middle School. After his educational journey at HCISD, he pursued a Bachelor of Science degree at Texas A&M University, College Station, from where he graduated in 1998.

Upon completion of his undergraduate degree, Dr. Muñiz gained valuable insights into employee management and the significance of consistent systems while working at Kroger Manufacturing in Fort Worth, TX. His pursuit of higher education continued with an MBA from St. Mary's University in 2002.

Following his graduation, he moved to Columbus, OH, to join Abbott Laboratories. During his tenure as a production supervisor, Dr. Muñiz developed a keen understanding of workflow management. It was during his time in Columbus that he identified his true calling, leading him to embrace his aspiration of becoming a pharmacist.

In 2004, Dr. Muñiz moved to Houston to study pharmacy at Texas Southern University. It was here that he met his future wife, Amy. After their graduation from TSU, the couple returned to Harlingen and began their life together. They are proud parents of four lovely children - Sophia Amor, John Robert, Patrick Robert, and Ariel, all of whom have inherited their parents' passion for music, dancing, and familial bond.

Dr. Muñiz currently holds a key role in his family business as the co-owner of Muñiz Rio Grande Pharmacy, a respected establishment serving the Harlingen community for over four decades. He is also the owner and Head Coach of Training For Warriors Harlingen, demonstrating his dedication to both his profession and his community.

Bobby's newest book, "Hormone Secrets: Decoding the Hidden Messages of Your Body," goes into much more details and provides the exact blueprint for living the peaceful, enjoyable, and stress-free life you deserve. You can grab his book for yourself at **https://www.drbobbymuniz.com/Hormone-Secrets**.

Empowering Women: Fitness Secrets for Navigating Menopausal Transition Successfully

By: Ava Gruszka

Entering the realms of the menopausal transition can feel like embarking on a very daunting and uncharted adventure. The menopausal transition incorporates the time period of peri-menopause (when hormones begin to shift toward menopause) into the years and even decades of post-menopause (the time after the final onset of a woman's last menstrual cycle). These transitional stages in a woman's life are most notably associated with physiological changes involving hormones, and metabolism. But may also incorporate a tidy sum of very serious life changes as well, like becoming an empty nester; parents aging or passing away; changes in personal relationships (divorce/re-marriage, etc.). Whilst this journey comes with its challenges and may feel like the world has turned on its head, it can also be regarded as a period ripe with opportunities for empowerment, renewal and reinvention! And fitness plays a pivotal role in this transformation. In this chapter, we will explore fitness and wellness strategies that can help you navigate this midlife transition successfully, empowering you to embrace this new chapter with confidence and vitality, and moreover regain some control over the uncertainty surrounding this new stage of your life.

One last thing to be noted before we begin - the fitness and lifestyle changes discussed in this chapter are meant to help women regain control over their lives, build strength and resilience, and help to manage the symptoms and effects of menopause. Fitness strategies are not a cure-all to the effects of menopause. In other words, you cannot "out-fitness menopause", there is no magic bullet. There are only strategies and methodologies that help manage, and deal with whatever has been dealt out. Also, there is no cookie-cutter, one-size-fits-all exercise prescription for the menopausal transition. Although the majority of women suffer from many similar symptoms, like hot flushes, sleep issues, weight gain, and mood swings, there can be over 100 other symptoms associated with this change of life. Everyone has their own story. If you are truly suffering, there is nothing wrong with surrounding yourself with a team of experts, from fitness coaches, dieticians, physiotherapists, doctors, life coaches, and massage therapists, to your friends and family! Always remember that you are never alone on this journey, and everyone with working ovaries will eventually go through this transition!

Let's dive into a real-life story of a woman named Laura, who, like many others, had been struck by the challenges of the menopausal transition head-on. Laura's story serves as an inspiring example of how she successfully navigated the often-turbulent waters of the menopause transition; emerging stronger, healthier, and more empowered than ever before. Her commitment to a strategic fitness plan, coupled with a shift in mindset allowing her to embrace the changes in her life, showcases the potential for women to not just endure, but also thrive during this significant chapter. Let's explore Laura's journey in more detail, discovering the fitness strategies that helped her to regain control over her own life change.

Once upon a time, in a quiet neighborhood, there lived a woman named Laura. She had always been an active and vivacious individual, but as she approached her late 40s, she found herself facing some new physical challenges that she had never experienced previously. As a former professional ballet dancer, Laura noticed an increase in joint pain, particularly in her feet and hips. In addition, although her current diet and exercise regime had not changed at all, she began gaining weight around her waistline at an incredible pace. Last, she noticed that the change of temperature she was experiencing multiple times of the day, were not because of the weather. Of course, these were just some of the more prominent issues Laura experienced, there were others like sleeplessness, hair loss and mood swings to add to the pot. Perimenopause had crept in slowly over time and had now permanently moved in!

At first, the symptoms took her by surprise and confused her. She was unsure if the hot flush was actually a hot flush or just the temperature in the room! Was the sleeplessness due to stress, or was it hormonal? As her energy levels for doing ordinary things began to plummet, and she began to experience unexplained mood swings, she knew that something was changing in her life and her body. At first, she became angry at the betrayal of her body and her lifestyle. She had always exercised, made healthy food choices, and taken good care of herself. This was something else! This was out of her control. The first step was to accept that changes were happening, the next step was to educate herself on what was happening, and what she could do to mitigate the effects. Armed with all this new knowledge and the assistance of her doctor, Laura embarked on her new journey to navigate the raucous seas of menopause. She wasn't going to let these challenges define her!

Laura had always been a believer in the power of fitness, having maintained an active lifestyle throughout her life. She decided to use her passion for exercise to navigate this transitional phase with grace and determination. With a detailed plan in place, she began her journey.

Cardiovascular Conditioning: Laura started her fitness routine by incorporating brisk daily walks into her schedule. The effect was two-fold: the obvious exercise effect and caloric expenditure of walking; and the reduction of stress. She reveled in the beauty of nature, and the rhythmic pounding of her feet on the pavement seemed to wash away the anxiety that had become a part of her daily life.

Strength Training: Laura was no stranger to weightlifting, having dabbled in it for years. She now embraced it wholeheartedly, joining a local gym to focus on resistance training and progressive overload. With the guidance and assistance of a fitness coach, she began a program with lighter weights and gradually increased the volume and intensity of her workouts as her strength improved. Not only did she begin to reshape her body, but her bone density also improved, lowering her risk of osteoporosis.

Flexibility/Mobility and Balance: Recognizing the importance of flexibility, mobility and balance, Laura joined a nearby yoga class. The soothing poses and deep stretches not only improved her ability to move better, with less pain and more ease, but also provided a mental respite. It was during these sessions that she learned to appreciate the mind-body connection, allowing her to manage stress and mood swings more effectively.

Mind-Body Connection: Laura incorporated began to include short bouts of meditation into her daily routine, finding solace in the stillness and tranquility it brought to her life. It helped her center herself and better manage the emotional rollercoaster that often accompanied hormonal fluctuations.

Nutrition and Hydration: Consulting with a registered dietitian, Laura revamped her diet. She introduced more whole grains, more lean proteins, and colorful fruits and vegetables into her meals. Hydration became a priority, with her daily water intake helping ease hot flushes and keep her skin radiant.

Throughout her journey, Laura consulted with healthcare professionals to ensure her fitness plan aligned with her individual needs and any potential health risks. She also sought support from her close-knit circle of friends, who shared her desire for a healthier, happier transition.

As the weeks turned into months, Laura's dedication and determination paid off. She began to notice significant improvements in her overall well-being. Hot flushes became less frequent and less intense, her mood stabilized, and she felt more energized than she had in years. Her body grew stronger, and she developed a newfound sense of confidence and empowerment.

Laura's story became an inspiration to others in her community who were also navigating this change of life scenario. She shared her fitness secrets, encouraging women to embrace exercise as a tool for managing this transformative phase of life.

Laura's journey through the menopausal transition was not without its challenges, but her unwavering commitment to herself empowered her to thrive during this difficult chapter. As she reflected on her experiences, she realized that this period of change had become an opportunity for growth, resilience, and empowerment. With the support of her fitness routine and her determination, Laura had emerged from this change even stronger and more confident than ever before, a testament to the power of embracing change and pursuing a healthy, active lifestyle.

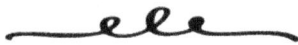

The Fitness Remedy: Strategies Unveiled

1. Cardiovascular Conditioning

One of the primary concerns during the menopausal transition is maintaining heart health. Engaging in regular cardiovascular exercise, such as brisk walking, cycling, or swimming, can help keep your heart strong and reduce the risk of heart disease. Aim for at least 150 minutes of moderate-intensity aerobic activity per week, broken down into manageable sessions.

Here's an example of cardiovascular workout incorporating several choices:

Before beginning any exercise routine, it's crucial to warm up properly. Spend 5-10 minutes doing light, low-impact movements like marching in place or gentle mobility exercises. Once you're warmed up, you can proceed with this sample cardio workout. Remember to consult with a healthcare professional before starting a new exercise program, especially if you have any underlying health concerns.

Workout Duration: Approximately 30-45 minutes (adjust intensity and duration based on your fitness level).

Equipment Needed: Comfortable workout attire and a pair of supportive athletic shoes.

Routine:

- **Brisk Walking or Power Walking (5-10 minutes):** Start your workout with a brisk walk around your neighborhood or on a treadmill. Focus on maintaining a pace that slightly elevates your heart rate. Swing your arms gently to engage your upper body.

- **Interval Training (5-10 minutes):** Alternate between short bursts of high-intensity exercise and periods of low-intensity recovery. For instance, walk at a fast pace or jog for 1-2 minutes, followed by a 1-2 minute slow walk to catch your breath. Repeat this cycle for 5-10 minutes. Interval training is excellent for boosting metabolism and cardiovascular fitness.

- **Dancing (5-10 minutes):** Put on your favorite music, or a favourite dance video from the internet and let loose with some dancing! Dance around your living room, incorporating various movements to engage your entire body. Dancing is not only a great cardiovascular exercise but also a fun way to relieve stress.

- **Stair Climbing (5-10 minutes):** If you have access to a set of stairs or a step platform, climb up and down for 5-10 minutes. This exercise targets your leg muscles and provides an excellent cardiovascular challenge. Use the railing for balance if needed.

- **Cool Down (3-5 minutes):** Gradually decrease your heart rate by walking at a slow pace or performing gentle stretches. Focus on your breathing and let your body recover.

- **Stretching (5-10 minutes):** Finish your workout with a series of stretching exercises targeting major muscle groups. Hold each stretch for 15-30 seconds without bouncing. Stretch your arms, legs, back, and shoulders to maintain flexibility.

Remember to stay hydrated throughout your workout and listen to your body. If you experience discomfort or pain, stop immediately and consult with a healthcare professional. Over time, you can gradually increase the intensity and duration of your cardiovascular workouts as your fitness level improves. Consistency is key to reaping the full benefits of cardio exercise, helping to manage weight, reduce stress, and promote heart health.

2. Strength Training

As we age, we naturally lose muscle mass and bone density. Combat this by incorporating strength training into your fitness routine. Resistance exercises using free weights, resistance bands, or your body weight can help preserve muscle and improve bone health. Start slowly and gradually increase the volume and intensity as you become more comfortable.

This sample workout is designed to be simple and effective, focusing on key muscle groups. Please consult with a healthcare professional before starting any new exercise program, especially if you have underlying health concerns and if you are unsure of technique, contact your local fitness professional for more advice.

Workout Duration: Approximately 30-45 minutes (adjust intensity and duration based on your fitness level).

Equipment Needed: Comfortable workout attire and a set of dumbbells (choose a weight that challenges you but allows you to complete the exercises with proper form).

Routine:

- **Warm-Up (5-10 minutes):** Start with a brief warm-up to prepare your muscles for exercise. Perform light aerobic activities like brisk walking, marching in place, or gentle mobility exercises for 5-10 minutes.

- **Squats (3 sets of 12-15 reps):** Hold a dumbbell in each hand at your sides. Stand with your feet shoulder-width apart. Lower your body by bending your knees, keeping your core engaged, and sitting back with your hips. Lower yourself until your thighs are parallel to the ground if possible, then return to the starting position.

- **Push-Ups (3 sets of 8-10 reps):** Perform push-ups on your knees or with your hands on an elevated surface (e.g., a bench or sturdy chair) if needed. Keep your body in a straight line from head to knees as you lower your chest towards the ground or elevated surface and press back up.

- **Dumbbell Rows (3 sets of 12-15 reps):** Hold a dumbbell in each hand, stand with your feet hip-width apart, and hinge forward at your hips, keeping your back straight. Bend your elbows and pull the dumbbells towards your hips, squeezing your shoulder blades together, then lower them back down.

- **Dumbbell Lunges (3 sets of 12-15 reps per leg):** Hold a dumbbell in each hand at your sides. Take a step forward with one leg and lower your body until both knees are bent at a 90-degree angle. Push back up to the starting position and repeat on the other leg.

- **Planks (3 sets, hold for 20-30 seconds):** Lie face down with your elbows directly under your shoulders. Brace your core muscles and lift your body off the ground, keeping it in a straight line from head to heels. Keep breathing, engaging your core and hold the position.

- **Cool Down (3-5 minutes):** Finish your workout with gentle stretching exercises. Focus on stretching major muscle groups such as your legs, arms, chest, and back. Hold each stretch for 15-30 seconds without bouncing.

Strength training can help you maintain muscle mass and bone density, which is particularly important during menopause. As you progress, you can gradually increase the weight, repetitions, or sets to continue challenging your muscles. Stay consistent with your strength training routine, aiming for at least two to three sessions per week, and allow your body time to recover between workouts.

3. Flexibility and Balance

Enhancing flexibility and balance is crucial for reducing the risk of injuries and falls. Yoga, Pilates, stretching and mobility exercises can improve your range of motion and stability. These practices also offer stress-reducing benefits, helping you manage the emotional ups and downs associated with hormonal changes.

4. Mind-Body Connection

Stress management is a key component of menopausal and perimenopausal wellness. Mindfulness techniques, such as meditation and deep breathing exercises, can help you stay centered and calm. These practices are not only good for your mental health but also for your physical well-being.

5. Nutrition and Hydration

A balanced diet rich in whole grains, lean proteins, fruits, vegetables, and healthy fats is essential during this time of life. Proper hydration is equally important. Drinking plenty of water can ease symptoms like hot flushes and maintain skin health.

6. Consult with a Professional

Before embarking on any fitness regimen, it's crucial to consult with a healthcare professional or fitness expert, especially if you have underlying health conditions. They can provide personalized recommendations based on your individual needs and goals.

Staying Motivated and Enjoying the Journey

Staying committed to your fitness routine can be challenging, but remember that consistency is key. To help keep you motivated and on track:

- Find a workout buddy or join a fitness class to make exercise more enjoyable.

- Set achievable goals and celebrate your progress.

- Keep a fitness journal to track your workouts, nutrition, and how you feel each day.

- Reward yourself with small treats or activities when you reach milestones.

Embrace the Empowerment

As you embark on this fitness journey through the menopausal transition, it's essential to recognize that this is not a phase to endure but an opportunity to thrive. With the right fitness strategies, you can empower yourself to navigate these transitions with grace, strength, and renewed vitality.

Remember, every woman's experience is unique, so it's essential to tailor your fitness routine to your specific needs and preferences. Empower yourself through exercise, prioritize your well-being, and embrace the limitless possibilities of this exciting new chapter in your life. You've got this!

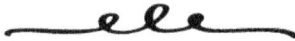

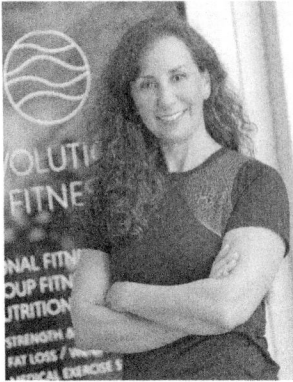

Meet Ava Gruszka, fitness expert, entrepreneur, dancer/performer, wife, and most importantly mom! With over three decades of unwavering dedication to the fitness industry, Ava stands as a seasoned professional in the realm of fitness and wellness. Originally hailing from Montreal, Canada, Ava has been serving the community of the Cayman Islands as a fitness professional for the last 20 years.

Armed with a dynamic fusion of academic prowess and practical fitness education, Ava earned a Bachelor's Degree in Commerce and a Bachelor's Degree in Fitness Education. This unique blend of business acumen and fitness expertise has shaped her into a multifaceted professional, capable of understanding the intricacies of both industries. For over a decade, Ava has been the proud owner of Evolution Fitness in Grand Cayman, a thriving boutique fitness studio and hub of fitness and wellness. Under her visionary leadership, the studio has not only flourished but has also developed into a sanctuary where individuals can embark on their own journey toward personal growth and positive change.

As an accomplished Certified Fitness Coach/Personal Trainer, Group Fitness Instructor, and Nutrition Coach, Ava employs a holistic approach to well-being. She understands that true vitality is a synergy of physical health, mental resilience, balanced nutrition, and self-care. Her coaching style combines years of experience, expertise and education, along
with empathy and compassion, creating a supportive environment that nurtures growth and transformation.

Over the years, Ava's main interest lay in the medical side of fitness. Helping her clients bounce back from injuries, surgeries, or illness. Recently, over the last 4 years, Ava has shifted much of her focus towards a demographic very dear to her heart - women in midlife and helping them transition through this new part of life and unlock their full potential. Fueled by an unwavering conviction in the transformative potential of self-empowerment and vitality, Ava has become an inspirational guide for women seeking to rediscover their own strength and embrace life's next chapter with vigor.

Looking ahead, Ava envisions a future where women in midlife not only achieve their very best versions of themselves but also revel in a life of confidence, happiness, and abundance. With her guidance, countless women have discovered newfound strength, resilience, and a zest for life! Ava is far more than a fit pro, she is a mentor and a partner in the journey of empowering women to live a more vibrant and fulfilling life! *"In life, nothing is certain; but anything is possible!"*

When Ava is not at work, you can find her chilling out at home with her family and her dogs; rehearsing for her next musical production; reading a book by the sea; or out brunching with her girlfriends!

www.evolutionfitness.ky

Conclusion
EMBRACING A LIFETIME OF WELLNESS

As we bring our journey through the pages of **"Fit For Life: Your Ultimate Guide to Health, Fitness & Nutrition"** to a close, we hope that you have found inspiration, guidance, and practical wisdom to set you on a path of lasting health and well-being. Throughout this book, we have explored the intricate web of physical fitness, mental resilience, and nutritional mastery, and how they intertwine to create the tapestry of your life.

Now, at the culmination of this transformative odyssey, we want to remind you that your journey towards a healthier, happier you is not a destination but a lifelong adventure. The principles and insights shared here are not meant to be fleeting resolutions, but enduring companions on your path to lasting vitality.

We've discovered that health is not a one-size-fits-all endeavor. It's a personal journey, uniquely tailored to your aspirations and circumstances. Your body is your lifelong companion, and how you choose to nurture and strengthen it will affect every facet of your existence. Remember, it's not just about looking good; it's about feeling great, both mentally and physically.

In the quest for health and fitness, setbacks are not failures; they are stepping stones. We all face challenges, plateaus, and moments of doubt.

But it's during these times that your determination and resilience will shine the brightest. It's okay to stumble; what matters most is that you get up, learn from your experiences, and continue forward.

As you move forward on your journey, keep in mind that health is not an all-or-nothing endeavor. Small, consistent changes in your daily habits can have a profound cumulative effect. It's about making sustainable choices that become an integral part of your lifestyle, not just a temporary fix. Embrace progress over perfection, and celebrate the small victories along the way.

Moreover, remember the power of community and support. Seek like-minded individuals who share your commitment to well-being. Surround yourself with people who uplift, motivate, and inspire you. Together, you can amplify your efforts and create a network of encouragement that fuels your journey.

Finally, never underestimate the importance of mindfulness. Your mental and emotional well-being are inseparable from your physical health. Nourish your spirit, practice gratitude, manage stress, and cultivate a positive mindset. When your mind is aligned with your physical efforts, you'll discover a sense of balance and fulfillment that transcends the physical.

As you close the pages of this book, know that you hold in your hands the keys to a lifetime of wellness. Your body is an incredible instrument, and with the knowledge and tools you've acquired, you have the capacity to play it with precision and harmony.

"Fit For Life" is not just a book; it's a call to action, an invitation to live a life that is truly fit for you. It's a reminder that you have the power to shape your destiny, to sculpt your body and mind into a masterpiece of vitality and resilience.

We thank you for taking this journey with us and hope that you will carry the wisdom you've gained here with you on your path to a healthier, happier, and more fulfilling life. Embrace this opportunity to be the best version of yourself, and may your life be a testament to the extraordinary potential that lives within each of us. Here's to your continued journey of being **"Fit For Life."**

Printed in Dunstable, United Kingdom

66132405R00131